THE CHANGING ROLE OF
MEDICAL STUDENTS

THE CHANGING ROLE OF
MEDICAL STUDENTS

Dr Jeni Harden, MA, MPhil, PhD, PFHEA

Reader in Social Sciences and Health, University of Edinburgh, UK

Director of Education, Usher Institute

Co-Chair of BeSST (Behavioural and Social Sciences Teaching in Medicine)

Professor Ronald M. Harden, OBE MD FRCP (Glas.) FRCS (Ed.) FRCPC

Professor Emeritus Medical Education, University of Dundee, UK

Editor-in-Chief Medical Teacher

Foreword by
Aviad Harramati, PhD

Professor of Physiology and Medicine

Director Centre for Innovation and Leadership in Education (CENTILE)

Georgetown University School of Medicine, Washington DC, USA

Ed Whittaker MBChB, BMedSci (Hons), AFHEA

Academic Foundation Doctor, Glasgow, UK

ELSEVIER   London   New York   Oxford   Philadelphia   St Louis   Sydney   2024

ISBN: 978-0-3238-7022-1

Publisher: Elyse W. O'Grady
Content Project Manager: Supriya Barua Kumar
Design: Renee Duenow
Marketing Manager: Deborah Watkins

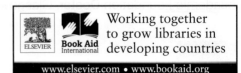

Working together to grow libraries in developing countries

www.elsevier.com • www.bookaid.org

Printed by Bell and Bain Ltd, Glasgow

Last digit is the print number: 9 8 7 6 5 4 3 2 1

Contents

Contents

Foreword

One of my greatest professional joys each year occurs at the annual meeting of the International Association of Medical Science Educators (IAMSE), where I have the opportunity to co-teach the *Essentials Skills in Medical Education* (ESME) course with my friend and colleague, Prof. Ronald Harden. Prof. Harden is an exceptional innovator and thinker and a world-renown leader in medical education who has helped transform education in the health professions across the globe. For me, our joint teaching over the past 16 years has been a treat, as I watched him inform, challenge and inspire faculty, students and administrators.

Each year, we consistently remarked to each other how the participants that year were interesting and engaging, and how we learned so much from them. Indeed, it was during these sessions that I first heard Prof. Harden articulate his views that medical students must understand the various roles they play as they go through the transition from medical student to resident and practitioner. In particular, he maintained that students should be actively providing input to co-create with faculty the substance, process and nature of their professional training.

After much thought, Prof. Harden decided to write a book, *The Changing Role of Medical Students*, with his daughter, Dr. Jeni Harden, a social scientist and highly effective teacher. Her experiences instructing medical students and as a director of quality assurance give her a unique perspective on the changing role of medical students. Together, this exceptional Harden team has produced a thoughtful and provocative book to challenge the conventional view that *teachers teach, and learners learn*. Rather, they assert that better learning will emerge if students understand the many roles they have as learners and take an active role in designing their own educational programs.

The book describes in some detail the seven roles of the student: *professional, facilitator, information processor, curricular collaborator, assessor, teacher and scholar*. Each of these is distinct, important and worth reflecting upon to understand, appreciate and optimize in order to create the most effective learning paradigm for health professionals. It also requires a conscious shift by faculty and administrators to empower students to take a greater responsibility for their learning.

The authors describe a range of student engagement in the education programme from little or minimal involvement, which is undesirable, to partnership and strategic collaboration, which is ideal, to having students fully in control of the curriculum, the latter of which is also not in the best interests of the school, teachers or the students. How to involve students and to what degree the collaboration is best helpful, is the challenge. I look forward to seeing how faculty members at different institutions and their student leaders strive to strike the proper balance.

The book also addresses the benefits of clarifying and encouraging these roles for students to engage in co-creating their education. The benefits extend not only to the students themselves, but also to their teachers and to the medical schools.

An interesting feature of the book is the chapter which provides student perspectives on these ideas, and perhaps is best captured by one who stated, "this book, in highlighting the changing roles of students, brings to the fore how students are no longer passive recipients of education, but active in shaping this education themselves".

In the Jewish Talmud (Masechet Makot 10A), there is a quote from a prominent Rabbi that reads: "I have learned much from my teachers, more from my peers, but, most of all, I learned from my students." This has been my experience as well, and I believe that it is one of the most rewarding aspects of teaching.

I encourage all readers of this book to reflect on the new and evolving roles for medical students and hope that the enhanced partnership between teachers and students leads to mutual growth and continued learning from each other.

Aviad Haramati, PhD

Professor of Physiology and Medicine
Director, Center for Innovation and
Leadership in Education (CENTILE)
Georgetown University School of Medicine
Washington, DC, USA

I am often reminded of Osler's famous quote when preparing to teach and am similarly reminded of it when reading the chapters contained within this book: "The successful teacher is no longer on a height, pumping knowledge at high pressure into passive receptacles." Though over 100 years old, this sentiment still resonates with the changes happening today. Not only do we see students increasingly seizing opportunities for their own learning but taking on roles within their institutions from designing curricula to teaching colleagues to pioneering research. Encouragingly, student doctors are often at the forefront of broader roles: activism and advocacy to create real changes to educational systems and issues that really matter to our patients and wider society. This book is a treasure trove of not only examples of these cases, but also practical guidance for educators and learners to use.

I felt more like a *passive receptacle* than an active collaborator in large parts of the early years of my university education (aside, of course, from the modules led by one of this book's authors!). My physiology and anatomy days felt filled with memorisation and parroting textbooks and lectures, with little else to my educational life. For me, this changed when transitioning from my pre-clinical to clinical education (or pre-cynical to cynical, as many of my peers would like to say) when helping to start a widening participation and peer teaching society. This opened my eyes to the issues of inequality in our educational system, but also to the fact that we, as students, could do something about it. Taking on roles beyond being a *passive receptacle* helped me to flourish as a learner. From here I became increasingly involved and excited about education, eventually co-chairing the Junior Association for the Study of Medical Education, a group of medical students and junior healthcare professionals involved in medical education around the UK. From this position, it has been a privilege to see that the roles of medical students are, indeed, profoundly changing for the better.

Dr Jeni Harden was one of my teachers at medical school, and in later years we worked on medical education projects together with other students. From my experiences and those I know from my peers, Jeni has proven an incredible commitment to student involvement in education. For example, through setting up an undergraduate certificate in medical education she has actively encouraged me and many other students to become more involved in teaching, assessing and curriculum design. Her father, Professor Ronald Harden, has of course had a significant impact on medical education internationally and on many students along the way. His earlier book *The Eight Roles of the Medical Teacher* quickly became essential reading for healthcare educators and supplied advice for their various roles and responsibilities.

The Changing Role and Medical Students will help educators and students see where learners' roles can be promoted to that of meaningful engagement and involvement in their own education. Importantly, many, if not all, of the lessons to be learned will be relevant to educators of all experiences. It is certainly not simply a toolkit for those starting out, but a book full of practical wisdom and novel ideas focused on those which apply to real-world settings. The chapters build up to a model or "ladder" for institutions to review, discuss and audit their own positioning with respect to meaningful student participation. Advice is given, for example, on improving collaboration between all stakeholders with a student-led working group, on educating the educators about approaches and benefits to student participation, and much more, culminating in an inspirational concluding section "Imagine if the impossible isn't". Medical students' roles *are* changing for the better, and this book beautifully encapsulates how and why, and how you can join in progressing medical education further.

I hope you enjoy it; I hope you find it as useful and thought-provoking as I have; and I hope its impact will be seen soon and for years to come.

Ed Whittaker

MBChB, BMedSci (Hons), AFHEA
Junior Association for the Study of
Medical Education (JASME) Co-Chair, 2020-2022
Academic Foundation Doctor, Glasgow, UK

Preface

In 1962, Sir Derek Dunlop, an eminent Scottish physician, respected by his patients and admired by the medical profession, wrote in the issue of the Scottish Medical Journal devoted to the Future of Medical Education in Scotland

> *It is important to remember that the actual details of the curriculum matter little in comparison to the selection of students and teachers. If these are good any system will work pretty well; if they are indifferent the most perfect curriculum will fail to produce results.*

Sir Derek highlighted the importance of the teacher and the student as actors in the education programme. More than half a century later, this remains just as true. Since then, much has been written about the curriculum and educational strategies such as problem-based learning, integrated teaching and learning, community-based attachments, the development of outcome-based education and assessment, including the use of MCQs, progress tests, portfolio assessment and on performance assessment instruments such as the OSCE. More recently, attention has focused on widening access to medical studies and the process of selecting students for admission. Less, however, has been written about and less attention paid to the key actors as described by Dunlop (1962) – the teacher and the student and the key roles they play in medical school.

In 2000, I (RMH) published, with Joy Crosby, the AMEE Guide "The good teacher is more than a lecturer – the twelve roles of the teacher". With Pat Lilley, I later published a more in-depth account of a teacher's important roles in a medical school, *The Eight Roles of the Medical Teacher* (Harden and Lilley, 2018).

The Changing Role of Medical Students shifts the lens from the teacher to the student and focuses on the different roles and the important contributions a student can make to the curriculum. We describe seven roles for the student:

- The student as a professional
- The student as a facilitator of their own learning
- The student as an information processor
- The student as a curriculum collaborator
- The student as an assessor

- The student as a teacher
- The student as a scholar

We describe the many benefits, both for the student and the medical school, if students are engaged in the implementation of the education programme. Working on their own without student collaboration there is a limit to what teachers can achieve. Working with students as collaborators they can do so much more. As Luccock (1955) stated, "No one can whistle a whole symphony. It takes a whole orchestra to play it". This text complements *The Eight Roles of the Medical Teacher*. The roles of the student and the roles of the teacher complement each other, with the recognition of a symbiotic rather than competitive relationship between the student and the teacher.

We believe that this book should be an essential read for all engaged with educating students. In *The Eight Roles of the Medical Teacher*, it was suggested that teaching can be the best job in the world or the worst. There are many factors that shape where a teacher may be on that continuum in any given moment. An understanding and appreciation of the changing roles of the student can help the teacher to see teaching as the best job in the world.

The seminal text on how technology will transform the work of the professions, including medicine, was written by a father and son, Richard and Daniel Susskind (2015). The Changing Role of Medical Students was written by a father-and-daughter team. Jeni Harden is a sociologist teaching within medical education, with thirty years of experience in higher education as a teacher, a curriculum developer and a director of quality assurance and enhancement. She brings to the book valuable insights and practical experience of involving students in the education programme. Ronald Harden brings his experience of over half a century as a clinical teacher, a curriculum committee chair, an undergraduate and postgraduate dean, a serial innovator in medical education and an editor of a leading medical education journal.

The book talks directly to the different stakeholders in medical education – teachers, deans and associate deans, curriculum leads, administrators and, most importantly, students. The relevant theory has been introduced where it is felt this will help the reader's understanding of the issues raised. The emphasis in the text, however, is to provide the different stakeholders with an understanding of the ways students can in practice engage and become involved with decisions relating to the education programme. Each chapter ends with a summary and key take-home messages.

In the first chapter, we highlight why students' engagement and involvement with decisions and activities relating to the education programme is important and we introduce some of the concepts and concerns that are explored further in subsequent chapters.

In Chapter 2, we introduce the seven different roles and provide an overview of the different ways students can be involved. In Chapter 3, we present the perspective of three students, giving their reflections on the role of medical students. In

Chapters 4–10, we discuss the seven student roles, as listed above. In each chapter, we outline different aspects of the role, present the benefits to both students and the programme or school, and identify potential challenges and ways to address these in practice.

In the final chapter, we look across the roles. The significant advantages of students engaging in the roles described are explored, and we offer advice on how the associated barriers and problems can be overcome. Guidelines and recommendations are suggested for implementing in practice, the roles discussed in the book. We present a ladder of student participation to help schools identify where they position themselves, where they might wish to be and how they can get there. Finally, we have highlighted the increasing importance of student participation in future developments in medical education.

In line with the theme of the book, as authors, we believed that it was important to collaborate with students in the production of the book. We worked closely with three students – Vishwani Chauhan, Anna Harvey, and Marina Politis. Vishwani and Anna are now junior doctors, and Marina is in her 5th year in medical school. Each chapter was reviewed by at least one of them, and their invaluable comments were considered in the revision of the chapters. Working with them on the book has reinforced for us, the value of collaborating with students. Their comments were insightful, often pushing us to think about issues in different ways and giving a perspective that would have been lacking without their involvement. A recent graduate and now junior doctor, Ed Whittaker also contributed to the Foreword to the book.

A wider group of students have also contributed reflective narratives in each of the chapters, bringing to bear a student's perspective on the chapter topic. We asked students to offer examples and reflections on their experiences. Students were invited to contribute to specific chapters or were given a choice of chapters, but we left the focus of their contribution open. We have not significantly edited their contributions because we wanted to retain the original intention and message rather than edit/suggest changes to make it "fit" or to illustrate specific points within the book. Rather, the students' contributions often caused us to reflect on what was discussed within the book and revise the content. These contributions are an essential part of the book, illustrating the breadth of medical students' roles, the challenges that students may face in engaging in different roles, but also the students' commitment to participation across the seven roles described in this book.

Throughout the book, we have used the terms "student" or "learner" and described the roles in the context of the medical school programme. Our focus is on undergraduate medical students; however, an understanding of the roles described is also of relevance to postgraduate medical education, the education of other healthcare professionals and to higher education in general.

In the title of the book, we use the plural term "students" deliberately to represent the heterogeneity of the student body. There is no singular "medical student" whose role in the education programme we can discuss in this book. Students enter and move through the programme with differing expectations, ambitions and concerns. As the student body becomes more diverse, students' experiences of the education programme and the roles they play outside of the learning environment also become more diverse. While drafting the book, we were mindful that differing experiences, responsibilities and persistent inequalities impact the roles that students may want to or have the capacity to participate in, and we have highlighted ways to address equality, diversity and inclusivity in students' engagement in the roles we discuss in the book.

Throughout the book, we discuss students' roles in "the education programme". Our main focus is on the formal curriculum – teaching and learning methods, learning outcomes, assessment and educational environment. However, the education programme is more than just the formal curriculum. The roles we discuss in the book also relate to students' participation in extracurricular activities that may be connected or independent of the formal curriculum including advocacy work, research and scholarship, and independent peer learning. We also include, as part of the education programme, students' involvement in decision-making and management within the school; the development of its mission and values; and the practice and policies through which they are enacted. Finally, the way in which the idea of student participation in relation to the roles we discuss is framed may reflect the hidden curriculum.

> The set of influences that function at the level of organisational structure and culture including, for example, implicit rules to survive the institution such as customs, rituals, and taken for granted aspects (Lempp and Seale, 2004).

Although our focus is on the changing roles of students, throughout the book we also refer to the "teacher". Medical education is distinct in that there are many people involved in a broad range of educator roles – university lecturers, clinical teachers, junior doctors, other healthcare professionals and patients. The student roles we discuss are relevant to all teaching contexts and therefore to all involved as "teachers".

We hope that this book will inform and inspire students, teachers and others with educational responsibilities to reflect on and be better prepared to pursue meaningful participation of students in the education programme with which they are associated.

References

Dunlop, D., 1962. Medical education in Scotland. Scott. Med. J. 7 (6), 245–249.

Luccock, H., 1955. Scholastic voice. Scholastic Magazine. 18, 89.

Lempp, H., Seale, C., 2004. The hidden curriculum in undergraduate medical education: Qualitative study of medical students' perceptions of teaching. BMJ. 329, 770.

About the authors

Jeni Harden

Dr Jeni Harden graduated with an MA (Hons) in Sociology from the University of Glasgow before taking on a Master of Philosophy in Soviet and East European Studies. She then began her career as a teacher and researcher, working as a Graduate Teaching Assistant while undertaking her PhD. Following several contract research posts, Dr Harden was appointed as a sociology lecturer at Edinburgh Napier University, where she worked for 11 years as a lecturer, then as a senior lecturer/subject lead for social sciences. In 2011, she moved to the University of Edinburgh to lead the social science theme in the MBChB and is currently a Reader in Social Sciences and Health.

Dr Harden has several leadership roles within the Edinburgh Medical School and College of Medicine and Veterinary Medicine (CMVM); Director of Education for the Usher Institute, Director of Quality (Medical Education), Co-Lead for Equality, Diversity and Inclusion in the College of Medicine and Veterinary Medicine. Beyond the University of Edinburgh, Dr Harden is Co-Chair of the network Behavioural and Social Sciences Teaching in Medicine (BeSST) and, alongside her co-chairs, has led several key developments in championing the social and behavioural sciences, including the development of the *Core Curriculum for Sociology in UK Undergraduate Medical Education*.

Dr Harden's passion and expertise as an educator was recognised in the award of Principal Fellow of the Higher Education Academy.

Ronald M Harden

Professor Ronald Harden graduated from medical school in Glasgow, Scotland, UK. He completed training and practiced as an endocrinologist before moving full time to medical education. He is Professor of Medical Education (Emeritus), University of Dundee, Editor of *Medical Teacher*, and was General Secretary and Treasurer of AMEE – An International Association for Medical Education.

Professor Harden has pioneered ideas in medical education, including the Objective Structured Clinical Examination (OSCE), the SPICES model for curriculum planning, the FAIR principles for effective teaching, the use of student portfolios for assessment, the Three-Circle model of outcome-based education, Best Evidence-Based Medical Education, and the ASPIRE-to-Excellence initiative. He has published more than 400 papers in leading journals. He is co-editor of *A Practical Guide for Medical Teachers*, now in its 6th edition, and the *Routledge International Handbook of Medical Education*. He is co-author of *Essential Skills for a Medical Teacher: An introduction to Learning and Teaching in Education*, *The Definitive Guide to the OSCE*, and *The Eight Roles of the Medical Teacher*.

Professor Harden's contributions to excellence in medical education have attracted numerous international awards, including an OBE by Her Majesty the Queen for services to medical education, UK; the Hubbard Award by the National Board of Medical Examiners, USA; the Karolinska Institute Prize for Research in Medical Education, which recognises high-quality research in medical education; the MILES Award by the National University of Singapore; the ASME Richard Farrow Gold Medal; the AMEE Lifetime Achievement Award; and a Cura Personalis Honour, the highest award given by Georgetown University, Washington, DC, USA.

He was awarded the Gusi Peace Prize for services to medical education and the honorary degree of Doctor of Laws by the University of Dundee.

Acknowledgements

We are grateful to everyone who has supported us in the production of this book. We have benefited immensely from the assistance of Jacob Thorn in the preparation of the manuscript. Thanks are also due to Adi Haramati and Ed Whittaker for writing the Foreword, which provides a useful introduction to the text.

We thank the students with whom we have worked over many years who have impressed us with the significant contributions it is possible for students to make to their own education programme. In particular, we wish a special thanks to three students – Vishwani Chauhan, Anna Harvey, and Marina Politis – who reviewed our drafts of each chapter and whose comments helped us to look at the topics from both a student and a teacher perspective, and inspired us to create an exciting and forward-looking vision as to how students can participate in curriculum organisation and delivery. They contribute in Chapter 3 their own perspectives on the many roles students can play.

As described in the preface, a wider group of students provided reflective narratives to each of the chapters, and we are very grateful to all the students for their contributions: Priyesh Agravat, Usama Ali, Emily Burns, Victor Chelashow, Alex Clark, Eleanor Cochrane, Vassili Crispi, Rania Fernandes, Katrina Freimane, Shreya Gupta, Siena Hayes, Molly Amira Kavanagh, Hannes Kruger, Helena Martin, Wesley McLoughlin, Catriona McVey, Rafia Miah, Vidya Nanthakumar, Callum Phillips, Simran Piya, Aya Riad, Arthur Sebag, Beth Selwyn, Margherita Vianello, Anna Wijngaard, Ed Whittaker, and Rumaisa Zubairi.

Finally, we would like to thank the team from Elsevier, including Elyse O'Grady and Supriya Barua Kumar, for their practical advice and encouragement, without whose support and assistance the book would not have been possible.

Models of education

Right now, in a medical school somewhere in the world students attend daily lectures with the lecturer talking on subjects such as the anatomy of the brachial plexus, the pathology of autoimmune thyroiditis, or the aetiology and diagnosis of Sjogren's syndrome. When not in lectures, students have tutorials, laboratory practicals, and formal teaching in the clinical setting. Preparing for the end-of-semester examinations they study their notes on a laptop. There are few if any opportunities for students in this school to be involved with decisions about the curriculum.

In another school, the situation is very different. Students have regular opportunities to provide feedback on the programme to teachers and course developers. This feedback is the basis for a continual dialogue between students and faculty towards improving students' experience on the programme. Following a discussion initiated by students as members of the school's curriculum committee, the number of lectures is dramatically reduced, and students have access to online learning resources designed to meet their individual requirements. To meet the needs identified by students for additional experience with practical procedures, students can arrange to spend time in the Clinical Skills Centre equipped with simulators and simulated patients. A mock Objective Structured Clinical Exam (OSCE) has been developed by students to help prepare their colleagues for the end-of-semester examination. Students also benefit from peer tutorials and participate in peer assessment, which assists them to develop their skills of self-assessment.

These two examples represent very different experiences and opportunities offered to students in terms of student participation in the education programme. Many schools are now moving away from the model of the first school and adopting a more participative approach, similar to that of the second school. Different terms have been used to describe the greater participation of students in the education programme including student engagement, the student voice, and student partnership.

In this chapter, we discuss these concepts, the context in which the move to greater student involvement is occurring, and the potential benefits. We touch on significant issues, which we return to at various points in later chapters.

Shifting student roles

Traditionally, the student has been perceived as a learner who studies, often though not exclusively at a school or university, intending to master a field of knowledge and acquire specific skills. From this perspective, the responsibility of the student is to learn; the responsibility of the teacher is to teach and facilitate the students' learning through the organisation of an appropriate education programme (Figure 1.1).

The past two decades have seen significant changes in medical education in response to advances in medicine and healthcare delivery, new educational technologies, changes in public expectations, and in some contexts, changing funding models for higher education. A move to outcome-based education and from teacher-centred to student-centred curricula has implications for the respective roles of the teacher and the students. Carl Rogers (1983, p 25) highlighted the changing dynamic between the teacher and the student and noted

> The shift in power from the expert teachers to the student learner, driven by a need for change in the traditional environment where students become passive, apathetic, and bored.

From this perspective, students were recognised as empowered individuals who can take greater responsibility for their own learning and for aspects of decision-making in the education programme. An example of this shift in thinking is the National Survey of Student Engagement in the USA which focused on

> What students actually do in their studies rather than what has been done to them by the institution in which they are enrolled (Yorke, 2014, p. xvi).

Within the context of these changes, the role of the teacher has changed (Harden and Lilley, 2018) but so also, as described in this book, has the role of students.

As a broad acceptance of greater student participation has become embedded in educational thinking, the range of concepts used to describe this involvement has expanded. Each concept leads to the framing of participation in different ways and may result in different implications for teacher-student relationships and student roles. There are often differences, for example, in the extent to which an outcome-focused or rights-based approach to student participation is emphasised. The former may see student involvement instrumentally, with a focus on potential outcomes

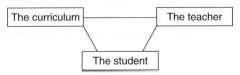

Figure 1.1 Attention should be paid to the role of the student as a key actor along with the teacher in the education programme.

that involvement can lead to. In contrast, a rights-based approach may stress the morality of involving students in their education. In the section that follows, we outline some of these core concepts – student engagement, student voice, student partnership – and point to some of the factors that have arisen in their development and application. This is not a comprehensive review of the subject, rather it is intended to give context to the roles we will discuss in subsequent chapters.

Student engagement

Student engagement has gained prominence in the discourse of teaching and learning and can be considered the broadest, perhaps umbrella term, related to aspects of student participation (Bryson, 2014; Lowe and El Hakim, 2020; Quaye et al., 2020). It has been recognised as a "hazy" term (Wong and Liem, 2021) and a "complex meta-construct" (Kassab et al., 2022). Some definitions focus on students' engagement in learning, whereas others suggest a multidimensional conception that extends to student engagement in wider school activities. For example, Groccia (2018) proposes a model in which

Learners can be engaged during their academic experience: in teaching, learning, research; with community, students, and faculty. Additionally, student engagement within these six dimensions can occur on cognitive, affective, and behavioural levels.

Others have linked student engagement with the concept of "active participation", which Bovill and Bulley (2011) note

Implies that students are engaged in an experience—whether that is university life, committee representation, or taking part in learning activities.

This is in stark contrast to the example of the first school, noted at the start of the chapter, in which students adopt a relatively passive role. Active participation requires students to engage in their learning and in the wider education programme (Meeuwissen and Whittingham, 2020).

This shift towards a more multidimensional understanding of student engagement also recognises that student engagement is inherently collaborative; it involves shared efforts and responsibilities, and the potential benefits can be felt by students, staff, and institutions (Peters et al., 2019). Nevertheless, there may also be differences between staff and students' understanding of student engagement. One survey found that students' understanding of engagement focused on the ways and extent to which they are asked for their opinions or are involved in decisions, whereas staff responses were broader, ranging from students attending lectures to the adoption of an approach that flattens hierarchies between staff and students (Headleand, 2021). There are many ways in which student engagement can be interpreted and so enacted. For example, Lowe and El-Hakim (2020) note the contrast between a "Students as Customers" approach, in which the focus is on course

> **Box 1.1** ASPIRE-to-Excellence (www.aspire-to-excellence.org) criteria for student engagement
>
> - Student engagement in policy and decision-making activities
> - Student engagement in the provision and in the evaluation of the school's education programme
> - Student engagement in the academic community
> - Student engagement in the local community, in extracurricular activities, and in service delivery
>
> *Source: http://www.amee.org/.*

evaluation and complaints, and a "Student Engagement" approach, which seeks to actively involve students as partners. It is this latter approach that is closer to the ASPIRE-to-Excellence (www.aspire-to-excellence.org) criteria for student engagement (Box 1.1).

The student voice

The student voice is a symbiotic concept to that of student engagement. Students, it is argued, should be consulted and influence the evaluation of teaching, the appraisal of teaching staff, student-nominated teaching awards, the appointment of new staff, and issues relating to governance of the medical school.

The student voice is often captured in end-of-course or programme evaluation surveys, for example in the UK National Student Survey (NSS) which collects information about final-year students' experiences and satisfaction. In this form, student voice is intertwined with performance indicators by which the school is judged. Evaluations are used as a proxy measure for teaching quality, and a catalyst for improvements, at the level of university, programme, individual course, and teacher.

The student voice may be seen as a simple sequential exchange between staff and students, for example when students provide feedback in a course evaluation survey and teachers respond. This, however, narrows possibilities for more collaborative, open-ended, and deliberative interaction.

> *Forcing complex educational issues into a 'you said, we did' model seems to strip them of the possibility for the serious discussion they often merit, with complex educational issues not discussed (Young and Jerome, 2020).*

To some extent, the concept of the student voice has become synonymous with systems of student representation. This raises questions regarding the authenticity of student voice in terms of the modes for hearing the student voice, the range of voices being heard, and the impact of student voice on practice. Within discussions of student voice, less attention is paid to voice as a right. The notion of rights is present more in the framing of student engagement as a "partnership".

Students as partners

The future of student engagement, argues Bryson (2014), lies in partnership. As we discuss in Chapters 7 and 11, the concept of student engagement and student-as-partner can be seen as an overlapping continuum of student involvement or participation. As you move towards partnership, there is an increased level of meaningful, active involvement, shared decision making, shared responsibility, and equality (Bovill 2020; Bovill and Bulley, 2011). However, while all partnership involves student participation, not all student participation is a partnership (Heeley et al., 2014). Indeed, there is often confusion about and inconsistency in the terminology used to describe student participation and partnership (Martens et al., 2019).

The Quality Assurance Agency Report (2013, p. 3) noted

> *The terms 'partner' and 'partnership' are used in a broad sense to indicate joint working between students and staff. In this context, partnership working is based on the values of: openness; trust and honesty; agreed shared goals and values; and regular communication between the partners. It is not based on the legal conception of equal responsibility and liability; rather partnership working recognises that all members in the partnership have legitimate but different perceptions and experiences.*

While useful in highlighting the values inherent to partnerships, this definition is limited in addressing the power dynamics that lie at the heart of partnerships, including those between staff and students. Hall et al. (2016), considering partnerships in relation to patients' involvement in medical education, propose a slightly different definition of partnership that is relevant to the discussion of students as partners

> *When two or more individuals/groups/organizations collaborate towards a shared goal of enhancing medical education, where one partner contributes something that the other(s) cannot provide… a partnership should have reciprocity at its heart, both as an ethical ideal and also a key driver for achieving positive outcomes, whether anticipated or unexpected.*

We return to these discussions in Chapter 7 when we consider the students' role as curriculum collaborators.

The move to greater student participation

A number of factors have contributed to the greater recognition of students as collaborators in their education programme (Figure 1.2).

Greater stakeholder involvement

The shift towards greater student involvement mirrors a more general move to involve stakeholders in the activities or work that relate directly to them, or in which they have an interest. In medical practice, for example, this is demonstrated by the move to shared decision-making, involving the doctor listening to, and working with,

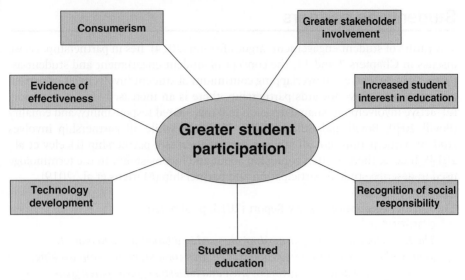

Figure 1.2 Factors supporting the move to student participation.

patients in their care. In medical and healthcare research, there is now an emphasis, and in some instances a requirement, that patients and publics are involved (PPI) at all stages of the research process. PPI is also now increasingly expected within medical education, with patients being involved in contributing to teaching and assessment, in consultations about curriculum development, and to a lesser extent in programme management (General Medical Council, 2009). PPI has also raised many questions about what strategies are needed to ensure that the involvement of key stakeholders can be meaningful and effective (de Bere and Nunn, 2016).

Consumerism and marketisation

The last few decades have witnessed the turn in many Western societies towards neoliberalism; reflected in higher education in the marketization of the sector and the repositioning of students as consumers, who in some contexts directly pay for the educational product. This raises questions about how students conceive their roles and responsibilities. During the COVID-19 pandemic, students questioned the maintenance of fees at the same level despite the fact that the education received by them moved from in-person to online learning. In this way, students' role in assessing the effectiveness and efficiency of the education programme comes in part from their consumer status and so in some contexts is integrally tied into the question of whether the programme delivers value for money. In medical education, consumerism has been reflected in students' demands for greater ownership of and responsibility for the education programme (Taylor and Parsons, 2011; Carlson, 2005).

Increasing student interest in medical education

Students increased interest in medical education is a further factor related to the move to greater student involvement. As recommended by the UK General Medical Council, teaching and learning is now prescribed as a topic in the curriculum and many medical schools offer electives or integrated degrees in medical education. The Association of Medical Education in Europe (AMEE) Student Essential Skills in Medical Education (ESME) programme has proved popular. Further evidence of the increased involvement of students in medical education is the increased number of papers on a medical education theme submitted by students to journals. For example, there has been an increase in submissions to Medical Teacher with students as an author/co-author, from about 1% in 2000 to more than 16% in 2017 (Harden et al., 2018). These publications include reflections on their experience as medical students, but also their involvement in educational innovation projects, some of which are student-led. Involvement in the education programme and the publication of papers relating to this may be considered valuable in that such contributions can add to the student's CV and may offer an advantage when applying for posts.

Recognition of social responsibility

Students are also now showing a greater interest in and awareness of societal and political issues such as sustainability, social determinants of health, and violence and are bringing pressure for the inclusion of such themes in the curriculum. Recently, students have been a driving force for moves to decolonise the curriculum, perhaps reflecting the increased diversity in medical student populations. This enhanced awareness and activism reflects wider societal changes and some greater diversity in students admitted to medicine but is also recognition of the accountability of medical schools to develop socially responsible doctors (Woollard, 2006).

Student-centred education

The past two decades have seen significant changes in the educational strategies adopted in the medical curriculum. In the SPICES mode of curriculum strategy analysis (Harden et al., 1984) a move from a teacher-centred to a student-centred approach is recognised with greater responsibility placed on what the student learns rather than what they are taught. This approach was designed to overcome some of the problems inherent in a more traditional form of education by focusing on the learner and their needs rather than on the teacher's input.

Other curricular developments now established in many schools such as longitudinal integrated clerkships, problem-based learning, self-directed learning, community-oriented education, outcome-based education, portfolio assessment, and the flipped classroom model embody and support the concept of greater student involvement.

Technology development

Fundamental developments in the availability of technology in education, such as the use of online question banks and virtual patients, offer new learning opportunities to facilitate students' learning and their engagement with the education programme. Online communities can connect students to wider networks: for example, female students can access women as mentors in specialities with few women via social media. Such technological developments have also presented challenges, for example in relation to professionalism and students' use of social media, and concerns about student engagement when students choose to watch lecture recordings online rather than attend classes in person. It is important to consider the ways in which the expectations of both teachers and students around educational roles and responsibilities may change in the context of new technologies.

Effectiveness of student engagement

A further catalyst for the move to greater student participation is the publication of evidence of the benefits associated with students' active participation in the education programme. Student engagement is often predicated on an instrumentally oriented belief that students' intellectual learning is enhanced when they have greater involvement in their own education (Astin, 1984), leading to greater academic achievement (Kassab et al., 2022). In addition, student engagement is argued to enhance learning through the development of wider skills including creativity, critical thinking, negotiation and collaboration skills, highly developed emotional intelligence, and persistence (Trowler, 2010; Pendakur et al., 2020). Student engagement is also considered a factor that supports students' psychological well-being (Neufeld and Malin, 2020).

Although our focus is on student engagement and the associated student roles, this is integrally connected to the roles and experiences of teachers. There is the potential for staff to experience their work as more rewarding when instructing students who are more engaged in their learning and working with students who are keen to contribute to curriculum development.

In addition to benefits for individual students and teachers, there are also wider benefits related to the potential for student engagement to improve quality assurance and enhancement processes. The involvement of students may lead to more authentic and effective quality improvements.

We discuss further potential benefits associated with student engagement in subsequent chapters and return to these in the final chapter.

Conclusion

Student engagement is high on today's agenda in medical education. We adopt a broad use of the term "student engagement" that goes beyond engagement in learning and includes active student involvement or participation in the education programme. The forms of student participation, the extent to which students have a voice in decisions, and the nature of student-teacher partnerships vary in different contexts. What is constant, however, is that the role played by students has changed considerably from their traditional role as passive recipients of teaching and education offerings. For students to be engaged in the education programme, potentially as partners and not just as consumers, and for students to have a meaningful voice in decisions about the programme a reappraisal of students' roles and responsibilities is required. The aim of this book is to describe the different roles that students can play in relation to the education programme. In the next chapter, we outline seven roles for the student that reflect opportunities for greater student participation.

References

Astin, A.W., 1984. Student involvement: A developmental theory for higher education. J. Col. Stud. Dev. 25 (4), 297–308.

de Bere, S.R., Nunn, S., 2016. Towards a pedagogy for patient and public involvement in medical education. Med. Educ. 50 (1), 79–92.

Bovill, C., 2020. Co-creating Learning and Teaching: Towards Relational Pedagogy in Higher Education. Critical Publishing, St Albans, UK.

Bovill, C., Bulley, C., 2011. A model of active student participation in curriculum design: Exploring desirability and possibility. In: Rust, C. (Ed.), Improving Student Learning (ISL) 18: Global Theories and Local Practices: Institutional, Disciplinary and Cultural Variations. Oxford Brookes University, Oxford Centre for Staff and Learning Development, UK. pp. 176–188.

Bryson, C., 2014. Understanding and Developing Student Engagement. Routledge, London, UK.

Carlson, S., 2005. The net generation goes to college. Chron. High. Educ. 52 (7), A34–A37.

General Medical Council. 2009. Patient and public involvement in undergraduate medical education. https://www.gmc-uk.org/-/media/documents/Patient_and_public_involvement_in_undergraduate_medical_education___guidance_0815.pdf_56438926.pdf.

Groccia, J.E., 2018. What is student engagement? New. Dir. Teach. Learn. 154 (154), 11–20.

Hall, E., Cleland, J., Mattick, K., 2016. Partnerships in medical education: Looking across disciplinary boundaries to extend knowledge. Perspect. Med. Educ. 5, 71–72.

Harden, R.M., Lilley, P., 2018. The Eight Roles of the Medical Teacher. Elsevier, London, UK.

Harden., R.M., Lilley, P., McLaughlin, J., 2018. Forty years of medical education through the eyes of Medical Teacher: From chrysalis to butterfly. Med. Teach. 40 (4), 328–330.

Harden, R.M., Sowden, S., Dunn, W.R., 1984. Educational strategies in curriculum development: The SPICES model. Med. Educ. 18 (4), 284–297.

Headleand, C., 2021. What does 'student engagement' mean to you? And you? And you? The Campus. Times Higher Education. https://www.timeshighereducation.com/campus/what-does-student-engagement-mean-you-and-you-and-you.

Heeley, M., Flint, A., Harrington, K., 2014. Engagement through partnership: Students as partners in learning and teaching in higher education. York HEA, UK.

Kassab, S.E., El-Sayed, W., Hamdy, H., 2022. Student engagement in undergraduate medical education: A scoping review. Med. Ed. 1–13.

Lowe, T., El Hakim, Y., 2020. A Handbook for Student Engagement in Higher Education: Theory into Practice. Routledge, London, UK.

Martens, S.E., Meeuwissen, S.N.E., Dolmans, D.H.J., Bovill, M.C., Könings, K.D., 2019. Student participation in the design of learning and teaching: Disentangling the terminology and approaches. Med. Teach. 41 (10), 1203–1205.

Meeuwissen, S.N.E., Whittingham, J.R.D., 2020. Student participation in undergraduate medical education: A continuous collective endeavour. Perspect. Med. Educ. 9, 3–4.

Neufeld, A., Malin, G., 2020. How medical students' perceptions of instructor autonomy-support mediate their motivation and psychological wellbeing. Med. Teach. 42 (6), 650–656.

Pendakur, S.L., Quaye, S.J., Harper, S.R., 2020. The heart of our work: Equitable engagement for students in U.S. higher education. In: Quaye, S.J., Harper, S.R., Pendakur, S.L (Eds.), Student Engagement in Higher Education: Theoretical Perspectives and Practical Approaches for Diverse Populations (3rd ed). Routledge, New York, USA.

Peters, H., Zdravkovic, M., João Costa, M., et al., 2019. Twelve tips for enhancing

STUDENT PARTICIPATION IN THE EDUCATION PROGRAMME

student engagement. Med. Teach. 41 (6), 632–637.

Quaye, S.J., Harper, S.R., Pendakur, S.L., 2020. Student Engagement in Higher Education: Theoretical Perspectives and Practical Approaches for Diverse Populations, (3rd ed). Routledge, New York, USA.

Rogers, C.R., 1983. Freedom to Learn for the 80s. Merrill Publishing Co., Indianapolis, Indiana, USA.

Taylor, L., Parson, J., 2011. Improving student engagement. Current Issues Educ. 14 (1–32).

The Quality Assurance Agency for Higher Education, 2013. UK Quality Code for Higher Education. QAA, Gloucester, UK.

Trowler, V., 2010. Student Engagement Literature Review. University of Huddersfield, UK.

Wong, Z.Y., Liem, G.A.D., 2021. Student engagement: Current state of the construct, conceptual refinement, and future research directions. Educ. Psychol. Rev. 34 (1), 107–138.

Woollard, R.F., 2006. Caring for a common future: Medical schools' social accountability. Med. Educ. 40 (4), 301–313.

Yorke, M., 2014. Foreword. In: Bryson, C. (Ed.), Understanding and Developing Student Engagement. Routledge, London, UK.

Young, H., Jerome, L., 2020. Student voice in higher education: Opening the loop. BERJ. 46 (3), 688–705.

The seven roles of medical students   2

Student participation and the roles of the student

Students' involvement with their education programme and how this may manifest is on today's agenda in medical education, as described in Chapter 1. While student engagement is recognised to be important, what constitutes student engagement is debated. The roles that students can play have not been prominently featured in such discussions. The answer to the question *"what is the student's role in the education programme?"* is complex. Students have different roles to play in the curriculum. Some of these may be obvious, others less so. The roles may also vary at different stages in the student's education, in different contexts, and at different levels (Bryson, 2014). In this book, we look at seven roles for the student and how the student has a specific function and responsibility, operates in a different way, and makes a unique contribution to the education programme in each of the roles described.

Exploring student engagement through the lens of the different roles played by the student helps to clarify the nature of student participation in the education programme, not just as a series of isolated activities, arrangements or mechanisms. Indeed, a consideration of students' roles contributes to a much-needed understanding between faculty and students of the nature and implementation of student participation. Engaging students as active participants in the learning programme requires the establishment of a culture where the different roles a student can play are understood and incorporated into the education community, with the partnership as something more than the sum of the parts, reinforcing cooperation, collegiality, professionalism, and mutual respect. While the roles described may be recognisable to both students and teachers, this does not imply that there will always be a consensus concerning the responsibilities related to engagement in these roles.

What can be gained from a discussion of student roles?

A consideration of the roles a student can play in the education programme can serve as a catalyst for considering the multidimensional nature of student engagement (Figure 2.1). It provides a holistic perspective and deepening discussion of what is expected of students in the context of a move to greater student participation in the programme. Exploring student roles allows the complex issues relating

11

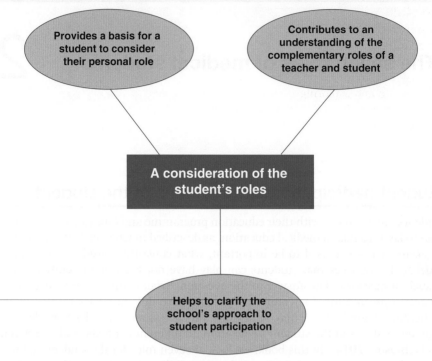

Figure 2.1 The impact of a consideration of the student's roles in the education programme.

to student identity to be considered; it is not just what students are doing and what is being done to them, but also what they are becoming that is made more explicit through the exploration of different student roles.

Addressing the roles of the student provides a language for exploring the different approaches to the implementation of student participation from the perspective of the student, the teacher, and the school.

Students

The extent and nature of students' involvement in the roles described will vary between students and over time for the same student. It is unlikely that a student will participate fully in all of the seven roles. The role lens provides a framework for students to reflect on their own personal contribution to the education programme and what facilitates or discourages their participation.

Teachers

As discussed in Chapter 1, there is a changing dynamic between students and teachers. An exploration of the roles of the student helps to clarify what is expected of the teacher, the roles of the teacher, and how the teacher's roles are complementary to the role of the student (Karakitsiou et al., 2012). It also identifies where there may be tensions.

The school

Some approaches to student participation are relatively common and widely adopted in medical schools, for example gathering course feedback. Others (for example, the student's role as a curriculum developer) are less common.

Reflecting on and exploring the student's roles is beneficial not only for the student and teacher but also for the school. Consideration of student (and teacher) roles can help an institution reflect on its approach to student participation, how the approach fits with the school's mission, how effective it is, and what challenges may be faced. We also recognise that student participation in the education programme may be challenging, particularly where there are tensions between the expectations of the roles of the teacher and student, or where there are barriers to student participation that may be beyond the control of the teachers, students, or even the school.

The seven roles of the student

We have identified seven roles for the student related to their participation in the education programme (Figure 2.2). These are described in the chapters of this book.

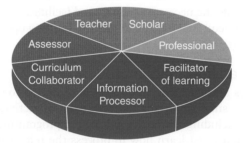

Figure 2.2 The seven roles of the student.

Establishment of the seven roles was informed by:

- A review of the literature relating to student engagement
- The practical experience of the authors as students, teachers, and curriculum developers
- A study of the teacher/student dynamic and the complementary nature of the student and the teacher's roles (Harden and Lilley, 2018)

The seven roles are:

The student as a professional

In medical education, demonstrating professional values is core to learning and assessment. The student must demonstrate professionalism through their behaviour and performance in patient care as a student doctor. This may be reflected in the Hippocratic Oath or its modern equivalents (Green, 2017). Students are also expected to show respect to their peers and other members of the healthcare team they study and work alongside.

Professional behaviour also relates to students' performance as learners: students should demonstrate integrity and honesty as learners. They must act professionally in their roles as digital learners, navigating the challenges posed by the blurring of personal and professional boundaries.

Increasingly, students' professional responsibilities are seen to extend beyond the individual patient to broader civic professionalism, such as in relation to the impact of health inequalities. Finally, being professional also relates to students' health and well-being and the shared responsibility between the student and the school for supporting the student's well-being by responding to and addressing related concerns.

The student as a facilitator of their own learning

Heutagogy places the student at the centre of their own learning (Hase and Kenyon, 2000). From this perspective, learners are autonomous, and learning is self-determined. The emphasis, therefore, is on approaches to enable students to facilitate and take control of their own learning and develop their own learning approach. For example, they may identify learning opportunities that match their personal expected learning outcomes. While this may be considered empowering for students, it presents challenges for the student if they have to accept their responsibility, and challenges for the school to provide the necessary support and facilitation. In clinical and other settings, it may be difficult for students to identify learning opportunities and manage their own learning.

The student as an information processor

The student receives an increasing amount of information to support their learning through lectures, small group discussions, practical activities, and the use of learning resources, including textbooks, e-learning programmes and open-access resources. The student must learn how to process the information available. The potential of information overload in a knowledge-dense and rapidly changing field of study such as medicine is a problem. Knowledge doubled in the 150 years from 1750 to 1900, in the 50 years from 1900 to 1950, in the five years from 1960 to 1965, and was predicted to double in 73 days by 2020 (Gilliani, 2000). Processing the information received is of great importance and students should use the most effective strategy. Even with effective information processing, the student cannot expect to learn all they require to know for a life-long career as a health professional. The practising healthcare professional must be able to find information to inform their practice as necessary, for example in relation to a new antibiotic, a change in a therapeutic regime for lung cancer, or amended guidelines for the management of hypertension. To prepare them for this challenge the student must develop the skills of an information seeker. As described by Patton and Friedman (2017), this requires the student to have the ability to ask the right question, identify appropriate sources of information, and evaluate the answer they find.

The student as a curriculum collaborator

There is a growing acknowledgement of the value of student involvement as collaborators in curriculum development in medical education (Könings et al., 2020). This role may entail evaluation of the existing curriculum through focus groups or surveys; involvement in curriculum management or review teams; or the co-creation and development of course content, learning resources, and learning approaches adopted. The benefits of students' involvement include greater student engagement and empowerment with enhanced motivation; improved quality of courses, with courses being more authentic and meaningful; improved understanding by the student and teacher of course aims; and the development by the teacher and students of education skills (Bovill, 2020).

The level of student participation as a curriculum collaborator and the appropriate level of partnership are likely to depend upon the context, the level of study, the relative experience levels of the students and the staff, and the attitudes of students and staff. Students and academic staff have different expertise to bring to the curriculum process, and there will be times when staff appropriately have more voice and other times when students may appropriately have more voice. Negotiating ways of working collaboratively can enrich staff/student relationships but, because it involves a significant move away from traditional relationships, can also raise tensions around responsibilities and expectations. There are also concerns about ensuring all students are able to adopt this role and that barriers to involvement are, where possible, removed.

The student as an assessor
Considerable attention has been paid to establishing best practices for assessment and systems of assessment in medical education (Norcini et al., 2011; 2018). Students have an important role to play in improving assessment tools, for example by providing feedback on whether the assessment is aligned with the course learning outcomes; and evaluating the coherence, purpose and range of a programme of assessment.

Students can also have a significant role to play in the assessment programme, through their contribution as peer assessors. This has been noted as particularly helpful in relation to the assessment of attitudes and professional behaviour (Lerchenfeldt and Taylor, 2020). Involvement as a peer assessor can facilitate students' ability to self-assess their own competence. Experience with self-assessment should be an important component of the undergraduate medical curriculum, and there is widespread advocacy for self-assessment as a powerful learning process.

The student as a teacher
The student also has an important role to play as a teacher and mentor. Peer teaching has attracted increasing attention and benefits both the tutor and the tutee (Burgess et al., 2014). In peer teaching, one or more students teach other students a particular subject area. For the student being helped, the assistance from their peer enables them to be less dependent on their teachers. Peer teaching provides new opportunities for students to enhance their learning. It is also of benefit to the students serving as tutors who at the same time may improve their own performance.

The student can also serve as a mentor for other students. This may progress from a casual arrangement between students to a recognised role for the students and the development of a closer relationship between the students (Akinla et al., 2018).

The student as a scholar

The terms "student" and "scholar" have at times been used interchangeably. The potential differences in the application of these labels raise interesting questions in relation to this role. Students can demonstrate scholarship in education by critically reflecting on their experiences in the education programme, applying an evidence-informed approach, contributing to innovating and introducing new approaches, engaging in education research, and communicating their experiences to other stakeholders through approaches such as published papers, presentations at education conferences and other events, blogs, and podcasts.

Emphasising students as scholars has educational and personal benefits. Students should be encouraged to use a scholarly approach when engaging with their different roles in the curriculum. The extent to which a scholar's role is encouraged will vary from school to school and is related to how the school values teaching. As a scholar, students can be part of a community of staff and students where scholarship is valued, with new approaches to education adopted and facilitated by student engagement.

Categories of roles

As described in the following chapters, each student role is associated with a range of experiences, activities, and responsibilities, has different characteristics and challenges, and brings its own contribution and adds value to the education programme.

The seven roles are in many ways overlapping and can be seen to lie in three categories (Figure 2.3).

- *Intellectual roles.* The roles of Facilitator of Learning and Information Processor have the overarching function relating to the development of the student's intellectual abilities
- *Governing roles.* The roles of Curriculum Collaborator and Assessor, while relevant to the intellectual development of the student, have the main

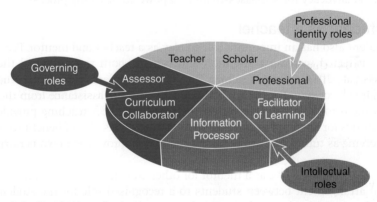

Figure 2.3 Categories of roles.

functions of governance and decision-making with regard to the education programme
- *Professional identity roles.* The roles of the student as Teacher, Scholar, and Professional are concerned with the professional identity of the student as someone who has a personal stake in improvements in the education programme

Conclusion

Student participation in the education programme is of the greatest importance. It is, however, a difficult concept as it may be perceived as challenging traditional approaches to curriculum planning, teaching and learning, and assessment. Problems may arise if there is a failure of understanding or even a disagreement between faculty and students about the students' role. For example, the institution's expectations of the student may be as a learner, with the role of the teacher seen as imparting the relevant knowledge and skills. This may be at odds with the view that a student can facilitate their own learning or that they may take on the role of assessor and improve their learning by doing so. Similarly, the development of the curriculum has traditionally been considered the sole responsibility of the teacher. The view that the student can serve as a curriculum co-creator disrupts traditional academic hierarchies and may be challenging for some to accept.

The model of student roles as described in this text offers a powerful lens to explore further the concept of student participation and how it may be implemented in practice. The seven roles of the student described above are examined further in subsequent chapters.

References

Akinla, O., Hagan, P., Atiomo, W., 2018. A systematic review of the literature describing the outcomes of near-peer mentoring programs for first year medical students. BMC. Med. Educ. 18 (1), 98.

Bovill, C., 2020. Co-creating Learning and Teaching: Towards Relational Pedagogy in Higher Education. Critical Publishing, St Albans, UK.

Bryson, C., 2014. Understanding and Developing Student Engagement. Routledge, London, UK.

Burgess, A., McGregor, D., Mellis, C., 2014. Medical students as peer tutors: A systematic review. BMC. Med. Educ. 14, 115.

Gilliani, B.B., 2000. Using the web to create a student-centred curriculum. In: Cole, R.A. (Ed.), Issues in Web-Based Pedagogy:

A Critical Primer. Greenwood Press, Westport, CT, USA.

Green, B., 2017. Use of the Hippocratic or other professional oaths in UK medical schools in 2017: Practice, perception of benefit and principlism. BMC. Research. Notes. 10 (1), 777.

Harden, R.M., Lilley, P.M., 2018. The Eight Roles of the Medical Teacher. Elsevier, London, UK.

Hase, S., Kenyon, C., 2000. From andragogy to heutagogy. Ultibase Articles. 5, 1–10.

Karakitsiou, D.E., Markou, A., Kyriakou, P., et al., 2012. The good student is more than a listener - The 12+1 roles of the medical student. Med. Teach. 34 (1), e1–e8.

Könings, K.D., Mordang, S., Smeenk, F., Stassen, L., Ramani, S., 2020. Learner involvement in the co-creation of teaching and learning: AMEE-guide no. 138. Medical Teacher. 43 (8), 924–936.

Lerchenfeldt, S., Taylor, T., 2020. Best practices in peer assessment: Training tomorrow's physicians to obtain and provide quality feedback. Adv. Med. Educ. Pract. 11, 571–578.

Norcini, J., Anderson, B., Bollela, V., et al., 2011. Criteria for good assessment: Consensus statement and recommendations from the Ottawa 2010. Conference. Med. Teach. 33 (3), 206–214.

Norcini, J., Anderson, M.B., Bollela, V., et al., 2018. 2018 Consensus framework for good assessment. Med. Teach. 40 (11), 1102–1109.

Patton, C., Friedman, C.P., 2017. Medical education in an era of ubiquitous information. In: Dent, J.A., Harden, R.M., Hunt, D. (Eds.), Practical Guide for Medical Teachers (5th ed). Elsevier, London, UK.

A student's perspective 3

Before we move to the first of the seven chapters where we explore the roles of students in the education programme, we present three pieces of reflective writing. We invited our three student collaborators to write a reflective piece about student roles, based on their experiences. The students read drafts of Chapters 1 and 2 and were aware of the roles that would be discussed in the book, but we did not direct them to discuss specific roles and we offered minimal comments or edits to their work.

Vishwani was about to enter her final year at the time of writing and speaks about her realisation that she would occupy several different roles as a student and that these roles went beyond the clinical and the academic. "This was the start of realising that even as a medical student I would occupy several different roles throughout university, and realising that these roles went beyond the clinical and the academic... I see now that in addition to a clinician, teacher, and scientist, a doctor is also an advocate".

Anna, who was completing her final year when she wrote this piece, drew on her experiences to reflect on the interaction between the multiple roles students have, both within and beyond medical school, and the identities that they bring and develop while there. She also notes the importance of educators being aware of the multiple roles students have. "The best educators I have interacted with, be that as formal teachers, coaches or mentors, have not only understood these multiple roles and identities but have also understood and empathised with the other roles and identities students might have outside of the academic or clinical space".

Marina was in her fourth year at the time of writing. She writes of the tensions she has experienced between her own interest in advocacy and activism and the medical culture that she found placed less value on such interests. "With students interested in advocacy and activism often written off as trouble-makers, naïve or both, I quickly risked becoming disillusioned, before my career in medicine even started".

All three students raise highly relevant and challenging questions about the roles of medical students that we explore within the book. As Marina pointed out, "this book, in highlighting the changing roles of students, brings to the fore how students are no longer passive recipients of education, but active in shaping this education themselves".

Vishwani Chauhan (University of Edinburgh)

I have enjoyed learning since I was in school. I would say I have been an information seeker throughout my time in education. Within this role, I have not only been interested in seeking existing information, but also in seeking information that we are yet to discover, in my capacity as both a "student doctor" and a "student scientist". This is perhaps one of the reasons I even applied to study medicine – I was fascinated by medical research, I wanted to learn more, I wanted to make knowledge and I wanted to apply that knowledge. I was attracted by the wide variety of activities that a doctor could do as part of their work. Patient-centred clinical activities, of course, but also teaching and researching. Having many different roles as a doctor was interesting to me as a possibility for my future career.

This was the start of realising that even as a medical student I would occupy several different roles throughout university and realising that these roles went beyond the clinical and the academic.

Like many of my peers, I went to medical school right after finishing high school. Professionalism in medicine was the first role that felt quite different to anything I had experienced before university. Even as early as our first year, we had the chance to interview patients in their homes and understand their narratives, which required us to uphold certain professional standards set by the medical profession and by society for medical professionals. Most professional standards seemed fair to me – communication, punctuality, teamwork, conflict resolution, and so on. However, many other professional standards seemed arbitrary. This was apparent, for example, from the #medbikini movement calling out a published paper that criticised doctors for posting photos of themselves on social media wearing swimsuits or holding drinks. The idea of the public image of doctors, in particular, is interesting because of its relationship with the way doctors perceive the public's trust in the profession. While *Good Medical Practice* (2013) outlines the importance of doctors maintaining public trust in the profession, what this actually constitutes can become complicated by society's biases, and medicine's own biases, against marginalised groups. From my experiences with my peers at medical school, I feel that younger professionals and students may be more vulnerable to this scrutiny, especially with greater use of social media. I have also found that marginalised groups are held to a higher standard of professionalism, as I have learnt from the experiences of my peers and mentors who are women, queer, nonwhite, disabled, and/or working class. This has also been shown by reports of BAME doctors being held to stricter fitness-to-practice standards by the General Medical Council.

The effects of these inequalities can be seen in medical education, such as the BAME attainment gap, which persists throughout undergraduate and postgraduate levels, with BAME medical students and trainees attaining on average less than their counterparts. In the wake of the 2020 Black Lives Matter movement, I founded BAME Medics Edinburgh, a community for medical students of colour in my university to find a sense of belonging. At the same time, I also surveyed over 50 of these medical students to understand the changes they wanted to see in their educational environment and drafted a 40-page report on this with the help of a 12-student team that I led. This spurred real change with faculty genuinely listening to the needs put forward by us students and setting up committees and plans to address these.

I had never seen myself as an activist. The idea of it felt uncomfortable. The reason I stuck with it was probably because the impact of what I wanted to achieve felt much more important than just "how this makes me look". My main internal conflict arose from the idea that activism did not fit with the image of the "objective" clinician-scientist in my head, the doctor-researcher I have aspired to become since before applying to medical school. A lot of my discomfort also came from medicine's culture of wanting to remain apolitical, which is a flawed effort, given that so much of health is determined by the socio-political landscape.

This experience expanded my understanding of the roles that I thought a doctor, or student doctor, should embody. I see now that in addition to being a clinician, teacher, and scientist, a doctor is also an advocate. In its most obvious form, this is as an advocate for our patients – "Why treat people and send them back to the conditions that made them sick?" (Marmot M, 2015) – with public health as a combination of prevention and social justice. But this advocacy also extends to how we as doctors and students treat one another and other healthcare professionals in the team. This means looking inwards to promote equality, diversity, and inclusivity within our community. This also means promoting humanism in medicine, recognising the importance of our own health and well-being as medical professionals, and having time to be able to process our experiences. These are not only crucial to our longevity in the field but also to our ability to connect with patients, as I have learned from the work of Dr Laura Vater, a haematology/oncology fellow in the United States.

Within advocacy, many of the principles of research and scholarship are transferrable. When I founded the group at my medical school, I applied the skills I had developed doing scientific projects throughout university – working in a team, conducting a literature review, designing protocols to gather evidence, and analysing and presenting data in a report and at local meetings. I learned these skills while conducting a lab-based research project on immunology during my intercalated year and again while doing clinical database research at the Edinburgh Cancer Centre during my clinical years. In retrospect, all these roles are interlinked; my capacity as a researcher helped me organise and enact change. The experience of scholarship gives doctors and scientists the skills they need to be advocates.

Although a recent revelation in my personal journey, activism and advocacy are not necessarily new to medicine. My medical school has a history of students who create change. I have lunch in the Jex-Blake Suite and Elsie Inglis Lounge. The women of Edinburgh Seven, Britain's first matriculated female undergraduates, fought for their right to study medicine at a time when the rest of the community wanted to oust them. Ideological conflict can cause tension amongst medics, who are firm believers. But we have come a long way since the 1870s. I have faith in my mentors and my peers to promote change in medicine. I applied to study medicine because of all the different jobs a doctor can do as part of their career. Now, on the other end of medical school, I am even more excited about this prospect. My definition of what it means to be a medical student and doctor has grown, and I look forward to working as a clinician, scientist, educator, and advocate.

Anna Harvey (King's College London)

I had a traditional route into medicine. Lucky enough to gain a place in my first round of applications, I accepted an offer to study at King's College London and arrived there the September after I left school, feeling pretty pleased that I hadn't been forced to take an unaffordable gap year. I had finished my A Levels with excellent results, had a barrage of school prizes and leadership roles, and had done hours of volunteering and semiprofessional acting during sixth form. While I knew that the transition might be tricky, with many warning me that it would be challenging to suddenly be "a small fish in a big pond", I was looking forward to meeting others who shared my interests. I felt prepared to go to medical school.

And yet, for the first two years of my medical degree, I was considered a "student in difficulty". I attended very little university, scraped through my first-year exams and failed the second year, and had to repeat my practical exams. I didn't feel that medical school was the place for me and planned to drop out after my intercalated degree in History of Medicine.

When I look back on this (rather unpleasant and stressful) time of my life, one thing jumps out at me as being the key issue as to why I had such trouble adjusting to university life: the fact that I struggled to integrate my existing identities with my new identity as a medical student, and potential future doctor. Communication skills sessions taught me that any personality, or deviation from the set framework of history taking or breaking bad news, was inappropriate and unprofessional. I felt unable to bring my whole self into my "performance" as a medical student. Objectivity was presented as a panacea; processing emotions was a distraction from the real work of rote learning anatomy and physiology.

This changed during my intercalated degree, where a handful of other medics and I were transplanted into the history department. The academic environment in the humanities is very different to medicine: students are encouraged to develop personal opinions and argue them. The academics with whom I interacted took an interest in their students as the classes were smaller and there was more continuity. We were encouraged to critically appraise our own existing prejudices as well as the evidence. After this year, I was much more secure in my identity and values and felt ready to go back to medical school and allow my identity to be visible to educators and patients.

In this book, we present the changing and multiple roles of the student and how these roles might practically exert themselves. What is less discussed, which I want to touch upon in this text, is how these roles might interact, and, more broadly, how they may come into contact with other roles students take on outside of the academic space: roles and identities that make them unique, that they bring with them on their first day at medical school, before any of these student roles are developed, and that continue to mature and change for a lifetime. It is inevitable that these existing identities, shaped as they are by the unique experiences of individuals throughout a lifetime, will impact the perceptions and processing of experiences during their time in medical school. To dismiss this and strive for objectivity in interactions with patients is to erase the humanity of students, and, importantly, means that issues of bias – both conscious and unconscious – are not addressed head-on.

The best educators I have known, whether as formal teachers, coaches, or mentors, have not only understood these multiple roles and identities but have also understood and empathised with the other roles and identities students might have outside of the academic or clinical space. As well as understanding these roles, they have understood the ebb and flow of these identities, which may be complementary or, sometimes, conflicting. Some days, it might be more important that your student is a child, sibling, partner, or friend than it is that they are a manager of their own learning. A respectful educator who cares not just about the learning and professional development of their students, but also their personal development and well-being, should have a sense of these potential conflicts and understand mechanisms of support they can provide when roles conflict.

Medical students are often (though not always) young people, who may be separated from their usual support systems for the first time. They may be far from home, perhaps in a new country, surrounded by new people and experiences both in and out of the academic world. Supporting your students to explore and find congruence in all their multiple roles should be a secondary aim of any educator who works with medical students. It is from this congruence that students can become more comfortable with themselves, more critically evaluate their strengths and weaknesses, and ultimately become happy, healthy doctors. Of course, one size does not fit all, and this support and mentorship must be individual, but empowering students to understand their own identities. Understanding how these come together to make up who they are would be a good first step.

Marina Politis (University of Glasgow)

Someone who I consider a mentor once told me that "one of the nice things about medicine is that there is room for all the rebels, misfits, and activists". As someone who has never felt quite at home in medicine, unable to conform effortlessly to the "medical student" role like many of my peers, this was a needed motivator to reinspire my drive to find my own place in medicine.

When I started the clinical phase of our medical studies, a peer on placement asked, "Why don't you wait until you've graduated to be political?" With one harmless comment, this person encapsulated all my frustrations with being a medical student. To me, being a medical student is inherently political as we navigate the complexities of a stretched healthcare system in an increasingly unequal country.

Despite this, we are taught not to be too loud or too opinionated or too disruptive to many status quos under the veil of professionalism – professionalism which often, in fact, only acts to reinforce traditional hierarchies and power structures.

This book and its chapters focus on the changing roles of students. As it outlines the changes we have seen in recent years, it is also important to consider the fluidity of various roles, even for individual students, as they traverse different spaces. We must also acknowledge that our role as medical students must not always come first. This notion is perhaps an artefact of a system that encourages us to prioritise medicine and work above all else, including our health and well-being. We can also be activists and catalysts for change, or cooks and sportspeople, or anything else, before we are medical students.

One aspect of student roles is that of student engagement, which has gained an increasing focus on today's agenda in medical education. But what does being "engaged" as a student mean and how does it relate to the roles we describe? To some, being engaged may mean scoring well in exams and having an in-depth knowledge of the aetiology, signs, symptoms, investigations, and management of conditions. To others, engagement may mean involvement in advocacy, whether engaging in topics such as climate change, sexism, or racism, or advocating for marginalised communities such as people of colour, people with disabilities, LGBTQIA+ individuals, and beyond. Others still may find outlets in activities such as crafts or sports or may develop special interests in particular areas of medicine, manifesting their engagement with medicine. Importantly, any hierarchy between these different forms of engagement must be flattened.

Virchow is quoted as saying, "Medicine is a social science and politics is nothing else but medicine on a large scale". For me, this rang true before I even made the decision to apply to medical school. Growing up largely in Ireland, the referendum surrounding the eighth amendment (which granted an equal right to life to the mother and unborn child) coincided with my last weeks of secondary school. Conversations surrounding cases such as that of Savita Halappanavar, a dentist who died from sepsis following the denial of an abortion after an incomplete miscarriage, formed a part of our everyday. When a sports teammate had a pregnancy scare, reassurances that we'd pool together for a Ryanair flight immediately followed, the meaning implied. Simultaneously, as a German, I was raised with an awareness of the Nazi atrocities committed in very recent history, including those committed by the medical profession. My grandparents always vocalised the need to take collective responsibility for the past. Medicine was political, and the choice to study it seemed to remedy my internal conflict between whether I wanted to study a natural science or social science.

Much to my surprise, the medical culture, seemed to insist that the socio-political was secondary to the biomedical. With students interested in advocacy and activism often written off as troublemakers, naïve, or both, I quickly risked becoming disillusioned, before my career in medicine even started. In these many moments of frustration, the peers, friends, and confidants I have found throughout medicine kept me going, serving as a reminder that medicine is what I want to do, and that the medical sphere contains like-minded, passionate individuals. This highlights the important role of mentorship.

The case studies in this book explore the many, diverse, and ever-fluid roles a medical student can have, ranging from advocating for inclusion of the climate crisis in the curriculum to changing culture surrounding mental health to promoting an awareness of LGBTQIA+ health and beyond. My question is: why do these identities still come secondary to that of being a medical student? Can we not be individuals, with our own identities, who are also medical students? Is the reduction of students to medical students just another tool of professionalism used to maintain an a sometimes damaging status quo? I hope that this book can serve as a reminder of the changing nature of not just the medical student role and wider medical culture but, most importantly, the continued opportunity for change and the power educators have in facilitating this change.

While the metrics used to measure medical students' success may still focus largely on grades and extracurricular achievements reduced to only national leadership roles and the alliterative trio of posters, presentations, and publications, we are much more than this, and each and every healthcare professional or educator who comes in contact with medical students has the potential to show medical students that they are more valued than a decile or point score.

By engaging in opportunities to drive change or become involved with areas such as research or advocacy, this can both empower us as individuals and improve healthcare education and healthcare systems as we advocate for staff and patients. It is important, however, to also retain an awareness of the challenges that this may bring. Medical students already face significant demands; such engagement is time-consuming, leading to a risk of burnout. In activism spheres, we may see an increased burden on already minoritised students (e.g., students of colour having to drive decolonisation of the curriculum in their free time, unpaid). Furthermore, while the culture in medicine is changing, not everyone is on board with lending a greater voice to students, and as students speak out, risks of victimisation remain; it is therefore imperative that staff fully support their students.

By highlighting the changing roles of students, this book brings to the fore how students are no longer passive recipients of education, but active in shaping this education themselves. Medical education can no longer start and end with the technical and clinical knowledge required in a clinical environment but must endeavour to create doctors and individuals who are capable of engaging with and questioning wider societal issues, for it is in these issues that so much of health and illness is rooted.

References

Good Medical Practice, 2013. https://www. gmc-uk.org/-/media/documents/good-medical-practice---english-20200128_pdf-51527435.pdf.

Marmot, M, 2015. The health gap: the challenge of an unequal world. Bloomsbury, London, UK.

4 | The student as a professional

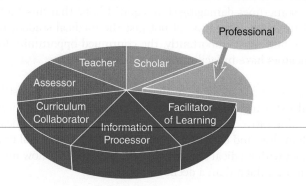

Students' professionalism

The first role that we consider in the book is that of the student as a professional. Professionalism is on today's agenda in medical education; the concept, however, may seem somewhat vague and be difficult to define, with variations in different societies and cultures recognised. There is wide agreement, however, about the importance of professionalism. In the AMEE Guide on professionalism, O'Sullivan et al. (2012) argued that

> *Professional values and behaviours are intrinsic to all medical practice, yet remain one of the most difficult subjects to integrate explicitly into a curriculum. Professionalism for the twenty-first century raises challenges not only to adapting the course to changing societal values but also for instilling skills of ongoing self-directed continuous development in trainees for future revalidation.*

Professional identity

Professionalism is related to the student's sense of professional identity; how a doctor or student thinks of themselves as a doctor (Orsmond et al., 2022). There are multiple perspectives from which professional identity can be understood (see Box 4.1).

> *[Professional identity] is heavily influenced by how medical students evaluate their professional roles and responsibilities in light of fluid circumstances and clinical experiences (Sarraf-Yazdi et al., 2021).*

> **Box 4.1** Conceptions of professional identity
>
> **Leedham-Green et al. (2020)**
>
> Profession identity can be viewed from multiple perspectives:
> - "Ideal": a collective contract with society
> - "Self and other": tribes and siloes
> - An expression of status: hierarchies and power
> - A coping strategy: depersonalisation and detachment
> - How we are seen by others: culture and identity
> - Contextual and situated: a sociocultural perspective

A student's sense of professional identity will, in part, relate to their personal beliefs, values and experiences that they bring to, and develop, during their time at medical school. They will also develop a sense of professional identity through a process of socialisation, learning shared skills, knowledge and ways of being. There are many ways in which the formal curriculum will influence a student's sense of professional identity, for example, teaching ethics and professionalism; opportunities for reflective practice; mentorship and role models. These can be embedded in the programme, in recognition that supporting students' professional identity formation is a core responsibility for the school (Sarraf-Yadiz and Teo, 2021; Gaufberg and Hafferty, 2021). However, the hidden and informal curriculum, reflected in the myriad of interactions with doctors, clinical teachers, patients, and other healthcare professionals that students will be part of or witness to, is also a strong influence in the formation of students' professional identity. While the formal, informal and hidden curriculum are often in synch in terms of their expression of values and expectations relevant to professionalism, at times there may be tensions in the messages students receive. For example, students may hear in a lecture about the importance of inclusive language when speaking to patients but may not hear such terms being used in clinics or may even hear a reluctance or rejection of such terminology. Students should be supported in navigating potential tensions between the formal curriculum and other learning experiences, but also between their professional and personal identities.

Four aspects of a student's professionalism

In this chapter, we discuss the student as a professional through four lenses (Figure 4.1).

- The student as a *student doctor* embracing the professional behaviours expected of a medical professional
- The *student as a learner* demonstrating professionalism in how they approach their studies and how they interact with colleagues and teachers
- Professionalism and the student's *health and well-being*
- *Civic professionalism* by which the student accepts a responsibility extending beyond individual patients to society more generally

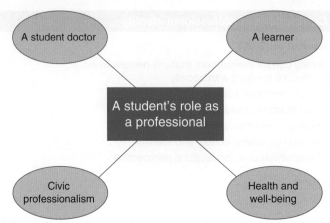

Figure 4.1 Four aspects of a student's professionalism.

Professionalism as a student doctor

Medical professionalism, suggested Sattar et al. (2021),

> is a central competency for medical students as learners and practicing doctors
> as life-long learners…According to the American Board of Medical Specialties
> (ABMS), 'Professionalism is a belief system in which group members
> ('professionals') declare ('profess') to each other and to the public, the shared
> competency standards and ethical values they uphold in their work and what
> patients can expect from these professionals'.

The General Medical Council (GMC) in the UK publishes guidelines for students
on "Achieving Good Medical Practice". The key features of these guidelines were
generated following a broad consultation with relevant stakeholders, including
medical professionals, patients and students. The emphasis is strongly placed
on the importance of a student's professional behaviour as a future member of a
"trusted profession".

> Your studies will bring you into contact with patients and members of the
> public, who can be physically or emotionally vulnerable. Because of this,
> and the fact that you'll be joining a trusted profession, we expect you to
> understand that there is a difference in the standard of behaviour expected of
> students on courses that bring them into contact with patients and the public.
>
> Specifically, your behaviour at all times, both in the clinical environment
> and outside of your studies, must justify the confidence that patients and the
> public place in you as a future member of the medical profession

Clinical placements
Advice on being professional in clinical placement is summarised in Box 4.2,
emphasising the importance of good communication with patients and colleagues.

> **Box 4.2** Being professional on clinical placements – practical steps
>
> From *General Medical Council, 2021. Achieving Good Medical Practice: Guidance for Medical Students. https://www.gmc-uk.org/education/standards-guidance-and-curricula/ guidance/student-professionalism-and-ftp/ achieving-good-medical-practice.*
>
> - Always introduce yourself to patients, letting them know your name and that you are a medical student.
> - When you meet a patient for the first time, check if they have any objections to having a student present.
> - If your medical school or placement provider has given you an ID badge or similar, make sure it is visible at all times.
> - Dress smartly and in line with dress codes set out by your medical school or placement provider.
> - Arrive on time for your placement and do not leave your placement early unless you have agreed to this with a relevant supervisor.
> - Attend induction sessions if they're offered.
> - Attend all mandatory training arranged for you while on a placement.
> - Make sure you know and follow the rules and guidelines specific to your placement, including how you should raise any concerns. If in doubt, make sure you ask if there is anything in particular you should know at the start of your placement.
> - Be honest with patients if you don't know the answer to their questions. Patients appreciate that you are there to learn.
> - Make sure you know who is responsible for directly supervising you on your placement and who has the overall responsibility for medical students where you are working. This will help you understand where to go if you need help and if you have any concerns you need to raise.
> - If you are not sure you are able to carry out a procedure competently, you should ask for help from a more experienced colleague, such as a nurse or qualified doctor. You should only attempt practical procedures if you have been trained to do so, and only under supervision that is appropriate to your level of competence.
> - If you think you are not being properly supervised on a placement, you should stop the work you are doing and raise your concerns with the placement provider and your medical school.
> - Always check with the patient what they have already agreed to in terms of treatment and they're happy for a student to be involved in their care.
> - Make sure your notes are clear, accurate, and legible even when made as part of the learning process as this will help you develop the skills you'll need as a doctor.

Safety and quality

As a professional, a student should learn about quality improvement and quality assurance and may have the opportunity to take part in audits. At the most basic level, the professional student should comply with occupational health policies and procedures in their medical school. Professionalism also requires the student to report any instance where things go wrong in the clinical setting or there are concerns about patient safety. Openness and honesty are necessary for their own performance, but so also is reporting the performance of others where there is a problem. However, reporting on safety or professionalism concerns may not always be straightforward. Johnson et al., 2018 found that students experienced barriers to raising concerns in terms of:

- Their understanding of when and how to raise a concern
- Recognition of the importance and responsibility of raising concerns
- Having the courage and resilience to manage the anxiety related to raising concerns

Recommendations from this research included improved teaching on raising concerns, clearer and impartial processes, and explicit support for students who raise concerns.

Ethics and respect

As a professional, students should behave ethically in all aspects of their clinical work, demonstrating integrity and adherence to the law in the application of core ethical principles. Beyond adhering to core principles and legal requirements, ethical behaviour also refers to respectful ways of engaging with patients and colleagues. Respect for the patient may mean admitting a lack of knowledge or capability or apologising if a mistake has been made. This not only demonstrates respect for the patient but also humility as a learner. Students must treat patients with respect by listening to and valuing their experiences and learning to work with them in partnership. It can be useful for students to reflect on their own values and judgements as they gain experience in clinical settings so that they become more aware of when potential bias leads to subtle or explicit forms of discrimination.

Such respect should also be shown to other healthcare professionals and peers. Students must be supported in understanding when their actions may be problematic or discriminatory. Many schools now run sessions for students to help raise awareness of unconscious bias, discrimination, and microaggressions. It is also important to offer students practical strategies to respond to instances of lack of respect or discrimination that they may witness (from a peer or other healthcare professional). Active bystander training may be useful (York et al., 2021), but adopting the role of an active bystander is not always easy for students, particularly when it involves a senior colleague. It is also important to ensure that appropriate, confidential lines of reporting are available to students and that students are aware of them.

Medical students must learn to work within teams involving different professionals. It is important for students to gain an understanding of the roles played within multi-disciplinary teams and respect the experience that their colleagues bring. This can happen tacitly as students spend time in clinical settings. It can be useful to introduce reflective learning experiences, for example, having students shadow nurses or healthcare assistants and reflect on that experience. Many programmes embed interprofessional learning within the curriculum. For example, the clinical skills team at the University of Edinburgh developed an Escape Room game to encourage interprofessional learning and introduce students to the simulation environment (Close, 2019).

Outside of medical school

The student should behave professionally both in and outside the medical school.

> *Medical students need to behave professionally outside of work and medical school. This means [they] should avoid doing things that will undermine the confidence patients have in doctors and the public has in the medical profession (GMC, 2021).*

For today's medical students, the prominence of social media has increased the visibility of their behaviour outside of the medical school and has heightened concerns about professionalism. As the British Medical Association noted, "social media can blur the boundary between private and public domains" (BMA, 2020). Research has identified examples of unprofessional behaviour through social media use including, breaches of patient confidentiality, discriminatory language, images of intoxication, illicit substance use, or considered sexually suggestive material (Chretien et al., 2009; Barlow et al., 2015; Pronk et al., 2021). It is clear that medical students now have to work much harder to navigate the boundary between public and private. This may not be obvious to students as they begin their medical studies, and students should be advised on ways to manage their social media accounts. Discussion of case studies is useful for students to explore potential scenarios that raise awareness of the risks and ways to address them in order to protect their professional personas and maintain patient confidentiality.

Social media, however, is also a useful tool for developing professional connections and for engaging with social and political issues (we discuss this further below). Jeanne Farnan, University of Chicago Pritzker School of Medicine, noted that the intention should not be to silence medical students.

> *Our students are super active in issues around social justice. We don't want to come at this conversation with 'The 10 Commandments of Facebook.' We just want them to recognize there can be consequences for what they post (Kalter, 2019).*

Professionalism as a learner

Professional behaviour as a learner

In addition to professionalism as a student doctor, a second area where a student should demonstrate professionalism is as a learner. The professional student has a good work ethic characterised by commitment, dedication, perseverance, and hard work. The professional student has a commitment to their personal development and continuing education. Examples of how the student is expected to behave professionally as a learner include:

- Meeting the commitments expected of a student as specified in the school's regulations. This may include any necessary documentation or photographic records. Students should attend sessions where their participation is expected and should turn up on time having completed the necessary preparation for the session. Staff will try to ensure that, where possible, sessions are organised in advance and that changes are notified and explained

- Accepting responsibility for their own learning, working to meet the expected learning outcomes for the course and completing assignments by the date expected. There is an often unwritten contract where the teacher accepts responsibility for the student achieving the expected learning outcomes and the student accepts the responsibility of working to achieve this. In the next chapters, we describe strategies that the student can adopt to make their learning more effective

- Accepting responsibility for mistakes and accepting feedback and constructive criticism from staff and peers, and responding appropriately with a willingness and desire to improve

- Relating to and communicating in an appropriate manner with colleagues individually and in a group setting. As noted above, schools can support students in understanding good communication and the impact of potential biases

- Working effectively in groups. Group work requires collaboration rather than competition with a willingness to help other students, share ideas, and contribute effectively to group work. However, there may also be a tension between professionalism as a collaborative learner and the overt competition of exams and job rankings that is apparent in some contexts. Indeed, students often express dissatisfaction at the behaviour of others who are "free loading" in group work, receiving a group grade while not contributing to the work of the group. It may be difficult to change the competitive context, but students' responsibility to their peers can be supported through professional teaching, and assessed through clear frameworks, aligned with professionalism criteria (McIntyre and Crawford, 2022). We discuss peer learning further in Chapter 9.

- Reflecting on the teaching and the education programme and providing feedback to the teacher and course organiser, as described in Chapter 7

An example of what is expected of the professional learner at Vanderbilt Medical School is given in Box 4.3.

Unprofessional behaviour as a learner

Students may demonstrate unprofessional behaviour on social media (Barlow et al., 2015). Unprofessional behaviour as a learner in medical school is associated with a greater likelihood that the student will have disciplinary actions taken against them when they become a doctor. Papadakis et al. (2004) concluded that

The demonstration that inadequate professional behaviour as a student portends poor professional behaviour in practice can now serve as evidence to some resistant students that they must commit to professional growth… we can now advocate from an evidence-based position that professionalism is an essential competency that must be demonstrated for a student to graduate from medical school.

Box 4.3 Commitments of learners as professionals at Vanderbilt Medical School

From *https://www.vanderbilt.edu/catalogs/kuali/som.php#/content/60da2185030bed95 0c90f815*

- We will respect students, colleagues, staff, and patients as individuals.
- We will strive for excellence in attaining the knowledge, attitudes, and skills needed for the highest standards of practice.
- We will attend all learning sessions designated as required by our programs. We will demonstrate respect towards teachers and peers by arriving on time, turning off mobile phones, silencing pagers, and complying with other specific expectations defined by the faculty.
- We will wear appropriate attire. In the classroom setting, our attire should not cause distraction. In practice settings, it should comply with the standards published by the institution.
- We will work effectively in teams, respecting the contributions of all members, assuming a fair share of responsibility, and performing leadership tasks with a sense of service to others.
- In practice settings, we will acknowledge and seek help if assigned a task that is beyond our level. If an assigned task conflicts with personal ethics, we will discuss this with the supervising faculty or staff member and strive to reach a resolution that places priority on the interests of the patient.
- We will recognise our obligations as a collegial community, sharing knowledge and assisting peers in their quest to achieve professional and personal goals. We will assist our colleagues in distress.
- We will establish the habit of critical reflection, acknowledge gaps in our knowledge, recognize our limitations, and strive for constant self-improvement.
- We will respect the intellectual property of others and will use online resources in a manner that is consistent with that respect.
- We will demonstrate honesty and integrity in all academic endeavours, including examinations, research efforts, and patient care entries.
- We will strive to create a culture of safety. We will accept responsibility for errors and near-errors by disclosing them, analysing them and implementing changes that would prevent similar events in the future.
- In the spirit of continuous quality improvement, we will accept the responsibility of constructive evaluation of our courses and teachers.

Unprofessional behaviour on the part of the student (for example, cheating in exams, plagiarism in coursework, sharing exam questions) will almost certainly be contrary to the school's regulations and may have consequences with regard to the student's progression. While such behaviour should not be condoned, it is also important to consider ways to support students in developing an understanding of what is considered "unprofessional" behaviour as a learner and how to avoid this. For example, supporting students' skills in note taking and academic referencing can help them avoid inadvertent plagiarism.

Professionalism as a digital learner

Students can now be described as *"the digitally enhanced learner"* (Ellaway et al., 2015), reflecting the increased use of digital media, including social media (as discussed above), learning aids (as discussed in Chapters 5 and 6), point-of-care information (such as drug databases and guidelines), or e-health systems.

> **Box 4.4**   Digital professionalism as described by Ellaway et al. (2015)
>
> *Digital media are not an intrinsic threat to medical professionalism. Professionals should use digital media for positive purposes in ways that support principles of patient care, compassion, altruism, and trustworthiness. Professionals should be aware of the shaping nature of their relationships with digital media, and they should maintain the capacity for deliberate, ethical, and accountable practice when using them.*
>
> Digital professionalism requires:
> *Proficiency:* the effective and efficient use of digital media supporting point-of-care management
> *Reputation:* maintaining an appropriate online professional presence and maintenance of the professional's reputation, recognising that what they do online will remain online indefinitely and refraining from disclosing anything that they could not defend
> *Responsibility:* accepting responsibility for actions on digital media, modelling appropriate professional boundaries for others regarding digital behaviours

A framework for digital professionalism is given in Box 4.4.

Ellaway et al. (2015) suggest strategies to promote digital professionalism around four dimensions that are useful for teachers and students to consider:

- *Awareness:* opportunities for students and teachers to engage in constructive discussion about the use of digital media should be encouraged. As technology is constantly evolving, these opportunities need to remain flexible and open to change, and students are often well-placed to identify such changes.
- *Accountability:* raising awareness can ensure that students are familiar with any school policies and regulatory guidelines relating to digital professionalism. Such sessions can also discuss responsibility and accountability when applied to digital media to address some of the issues noted above and promote the positive uses of digital media; for example, enhancing patient safety.
- *Alignment:* rather than seeing "digital professionalism" as a separate topic or skill, it should be *"woven into the fabric of the curriculum as a whole" and "folded into the ongoing development of competencies, milestones, and entrustable professional activities (EPAs)"* (Ellaway et al., 2015, p. 847). For example, the increasing use of digital media for patient consultations can be embedded in communication skills sessions.
- *Assessment:* to promote the alignment of digital professionalism with the curriculum, it is important to include skills that demonstrate this within core assessments.

Professional communities of learners

Students' professionalism as a learner can be enhanced by working collectively. Elsewhere in the book, we have discussed peer collaborative learning (Chapters 5 and 6) and curriculum collaboration (Chapter 7). Collaborative approaches can support students' development in their role as a professional. The significance of "communities of practice" (Buckley et al., 2019) is increasingly being recognised as a beneficial way for doctors to work collectively to share and develop evidence-based practice (Ranmuthugala et al., 2011). There are many ways students can develop their professional identity and belong to the medical "community of practice",

Box 4.5   Student case study: creating STASHH – the next generation of genito-urinary medicine doctors

A reflection by Beth Selwyn, Eleanor Cochrane, University of Birmingham, on medical students and a community of practice

The Student and Trainee Association for Sexual Health and HIV Medicine (STASHH) was developed in 2021 by Dr Hannah Church, Dr Eleanor Crook, and final-year medical student Eleanor Cochrane, with support from the British Association of Sexual Health and HIV medicine (BASHH). STASHH was created as a junior speciality association, to raise awareness of the GUM speciality and increase the recruitment drive to sexual health and HIV training programmes by facilitating clinical and academic opportunities for medical students and pre-speciality trainees. They provide educational opportunities, support career development, promote and facilitate research opportunities, and facilitate project presentation opportunities (Cochrane and Crook, 2021; Lim and Selwyn, 2021).

The STASHH committee recruited Medical Student Representative Beth Selwyn and Pre-Speciality Doctor Representatives Jason Lim and Hanna Nguyen. The preliminary task for these steering committee members was to provide near-peer representation and select local medical school and pre-speciality representatives for each of the medical schools and foundation deaneries within the UK, forming a network that can communicate our mission and activities to their peers.

For smaller specialities such as GUM, it is beneficial for medical students and pre-speciality doctors to feel part of a community, feel motivated by more experienced doctors, and to have accessible and realistic role models. It is extremely fulfilling and exciting to be involved in such a project, and we look forward to seeing the impact that STASHH has on the recruitment of genito-urinary medicine doctors.

for example, developing their medical students' communities of practice (locally, nationally and internationally) and getting involved in more specific communities of practice related to specialities or special interests (Cruess et al., 2018).

Boxes 4.5 and 4.6 present two examples of student involvement in communities of practice. In Box 4.5, two students reflect on their role in STASHH (Student and Trainee Association for Sexual Health and HIV Medicine), a group that was set up to support career development, research and education in genito-urinary medicine. In Box 4.6, a student reflects on her role as Senior President of the Royal Medical Society in Edinburgh, a society that aims to further the medical education of its members and build community among medical students.

Professionalism and the student's health and well-being

Student health and well-being is a challenge

We have looked in this chapter at the student's role as a professional from the perspectives of the student as a student doctor and the student as a learner. A third and sometimes ignored aspect of professionalism is the student's responsibility for their health and well-being. Well-being is commonly understood as a holistic concept referring to both physical and mental health and positivity. However, with the emphasis on acquiring the necessary knowledge and skills expected of a doctor and a focus on achievement and high performance in education, health and well-being has almost seemed like an afterthought.

Box 4.6 Student case study: communities of learners

A reflection by Simran Piya, University of Edinburgh, on her involvement in the Royal Medical Society in Edinburgh

Throughout my 5 years in medical school, I was mainly involved as a member of the Royal Medical Society in Edinburgh, a team of 14 medical students across different years who work together to promote medical education, student engagement and community within the medical school. I was involved with the society for 3 years, and it was in the last year that I took on more of a managerial role as Senior President. My main aim as Senior President was to foster an environment for discussion and innovation for the next generation of doctors. At first, this position was very daunting and a big challenge as it involved representing a society with nearly 300 years worth of history and reputation. In addition, it was a role with great responsibility as I was overseeing all events, managing and delegating tasks, and changing policies within the society to ensure everything ran smoothly and that members were satisfied. Nevertheless, this position was greatly empowering as a medical student. It taught me about managerial and leadership skills, teamwork, and the importance of professionalism.

Medical school can be a stressful and challenging experience for many students, and this has been exacerbated by the COVID pandemic (O'Byrne et al., 2021). Research with students in many countries has reinforced concerns that they are experiencing rising rates of anxiety, depression, suicidal ideation, trauma, substance abuse, and exhaustion (Pacheco et al., 2017; Farrell et al., 2019; Wilkes et al., 2019). A student's well-being is pivotal to their success as a learner and is fundamental to academic success (Scherer and Leshner, 2021). Well-being is also significant to the student's care of patients as a student doctor (Dyrbye et al., 2010; 2016).

Well-being should be a shared responsibility

Strategies to improve well-being often relate to lifestyle changes that students can make to improve their physical and mental health and reduce stress including changing exercise, diet and sleep patterns (Henning et al., 2018). It is likely that students will be aware of the benefits and potential risks to their well-being associated with these factors. However, it may be useful to embed simple messages to promote good practice at key points. For example, when students are considering the impact on their patient's health, they could be encouraged to reflect on their own practice.

Mindfulness-based interventions have received a lot of attention in recent years as a method of reducing stress and depression and improving the well-being of students (Daya and Hearn, 2018).

[Mind-body skills] focus attention on the relationship between the brain, mind, and body through specific techniques such as meditation, relaxation, and guided imagery to affect psychological and physiological functioning" (Saunders et al., 2007).

Mind-body medicine training can be beneficial to students but may also have a long-term positive impact on physicians in terms of their personal care and how they approach patient care (Staffaroni et al., 2017).

While there is a clear benefit to be gained from mindfulness training and changes to lifestyle, the school must create conditions and an environment where the problem of student well-being is addressed, and the necessary support system is available. Concerned about the poor mental health of their students, Stuart Slavin, the then Dean for Curriculum at Saint Louis University School of Medicine, United States, initiated the development of a well-being model. He understood that the problems with well-being lay more with the learning environment than the students' behaviour and a key feature of the model was to "reduce unnecessary stressors and enhance the learning environment". Changes to the pre-clerkship years included a change from a four-tier to a two-tier (pass/fail) grading system, a reduction of curriculum hours in all courses by 10% and a reduction in the amount of detail taught (Slavin, 2019).

Reflecting on the changes introduced over a decade, Slavin noted that

> Our initial goal was to improve students' well-being, but I now believe that we accomplished much more, and from that, well-being ensued. Students felt listened to, valued, and respected. They found purpose and meaning. They grew not just as future doctors but as people. I firmly believe that the same is possible elsewhere (Slavin, 2019, p. 774).

In addition to changes to the learning environment, schools can also support students' well-being by adequately resourcing support services; involving students in the development of support services to ensure they are fit for purpose; and offering financial support for students experiencing hardship. Such measures ensure that the challenges that can negatively impact students' well-being can be addressed in appropriate ways. The goal of improving student mental well-being can only be achieved through an effective partnership between students and institutional actors (Baik et al., 2019). Students must take a measure of responsibility and engage actively as participants in a well-being and health programme, but the school should listen to the voice and perspectives of students and be prepared to make radical changes if required in order to address the factors that are barriers to improving student well-being.

Civic professionalism

What is civic professionalism?

Considered less often but nonetheless important when considering a student's role as a professional is their civic professionalism. Civic professionalism is associated with the student's social responsibilities with regard to issues such as sustainability, inequalities, and gun violence. The UNESCO report *"Thinking Higher and Beyond: Perspectives and Futures of Higher Education in 2050"* (2021) argues that

> Values such as respect, empathy, equality, and solidarity should be at the core of future HEIs [Higher Education Institutions] and their missions. In other words, 'education with a soul' that 'prepares learners not only for livelihood but for life'…supporting them 'to be better citizens, more aware of their civic and environmental responsibilities'.

Civic professionalism lies at the intersection of formal knowledge and practical skills and a commitment to the common good (Koritz and Schadewald, 2015).

> *In this model, knowledge, practice, and the common good co-define and cross-fertilize each other. Knowledge becomes a necessarily integrative pursuit, work becomes a path toward individual and communal flourishing, and civic responsibility becomes a continual aim.*

In medical education, civic professionalism requires a sense of responsibility for the good of society, not just for the individual patient.

Unlike the concept of the student's professionalism as a doctor or learner, civic professionalism has not been crystalised and is open for debate as to the form it should take and the terms of action or advocacy.

How can schools support civic professionalism?

Many students are involved in extracurricular work that both demonstrates and deepens their civic professionalism. In Chapter 7, we noted that students are often the agents for change in the curriculum with respect to highlighting the needs of specific populations. As an excellent example of such work, in Box 4.7 a student reflects on *Amar Doctor*, a health education initiative she set up for immigrant Bangladeshi women. However, it is important to remember that not all students are in a position to engage in extracurricular work. We have raised this issue in several other chapters; the need to ensure equity in participation in many of the roles we describe in this book. In Box 4.8 a student reflects on his role as a minority advocate, the "duty" that he feels to help people, but also the emotional and financial challenges of doing so. He argues that "it's beyond time that [advocacy work] is recognised".

While deeply impressive work such as this is, medical schools should not rely on the development of civic professionalism through committed students' extra-curricular activities. The civic professionalism of students is directly connected to the social responsibility of the medical school in meeting its obligations to the community it serves (local, national or global). Schools should consider how they are currently supporting students to become socially responsible graduates. Some examples of good practice can be seen among the schools awarded the ASPIRE to Excellence Social Accountability award (http://aspire-to-excellence.org/Areas±of±Excellence).

In an analysis of the optimum forms of professional education, Sullivan and Benner (2005) highlight education that uses the clinical programme, mentoring by practitioners, and ethical reflection to provide students with the academic knowledge, practical skills, and "educated conscience" as the basis of an identity as a "civic professional". The education programme should provide the student not only with the knowledge and skills to function as a doctor responsible for the management of individual patients but also an understanding and commitment to bring their training to bear on specific circumstances which best serve the community. This

Box 4.7 Student case study: Amar Doctor: a health education initiative

An example of civic professionalism by Rafia Miah, University Hospitals Birmingham

There are many ethnic minority populations that make up the United Kingdom, each with its own cultural traits and health profiles. This presents a complex challenge to healthcare professionals in terms of access and to provision for good healthcare. In August 2020, Public Health England reported that Bangladeshis were at the highest risk of dying from coronavirus. In fact, Bangladeshis in the UK are associated with high levels of child poverty, overcrowding, unemployment, chronic health conditions, and long-term disability. Bangladeshi women are one of the most underserved communities with the poorest health outcomes in the UK. This is due to a number of factors including language, digital literacy, cultural stigma, and lack of confidence.

As a Bangladeshi myself, I find it difficult to comprehend that our parents have immigrated here for better educational opportunities at the expense of their own health and comfort. In response to this, I set up *Amar Doctor* – meaning "my doctor" in my mother tongue Bangla – a health education initiative for immigrant Bangladeshi women.

Amar Doctor aims to tackle barriers that Bangladeshi women face when accessing health education. We designed a series of six evidence-based workshops, covering key topics in women's health including mental health, breast cancer, and vaccine hesitancy. These sessions were delivered in a secure online seminar format via Zoom. They were delivered in Bangla by female health professionals and were open to women worldwide. We conducted surveys before and after each workshop to evaluate the impact of our intervention. Understanding the health beliefs, practices, and cultural needs of patients from different backgrounds is essential to delivering good healthcare to diverse populations.

Box 4.8 Student case study: the medical student as the [unpaid] advocate

A reflection on the benefits and challenges of advocacy work, by Callum Phillips, University of Southampton

We should be encouraged to be advocates – many of us already are. We want to help people and are put in situations where we confront inequity. As a minority student, I feel it is my duty. We have a powerful voice, hence why so many people want to utilise it. I am incredibly proud of the advocacy work I have done alongside my studies. I have created podcasts, written articles, and produced extensive amounts of content – including the design, editing, and curation of a dedicated LGBTQ+ issue of the British Student Doctor Journal. I sit on the committee of the Association of LGBTQ+ Doctors and Dentists, and I am a representative at meetings of the Coalition against Conversion Therapy, amongst other things. All this involves expending cognitive and emotional labour, shouldering the work of educating my heteronormative teachers and peers, and legitimising people like me in medicine. I have received lovely messages from the most surprising sources about how they've been helped by my work.

We should also be recognised for this work – we do things people have full-time jobs to do. This is especially true of minoritised students who, alongside these average expectations, have their trauma capitalised on to educate the very systems and people inflicting it. The extent of our acknowledgement should not be a certificate 5 years down the line to display our "leadership skills".

Being a medical student and a minority advocate does not come cheap; it is beyond time that fact is recognised.

> **Box 4.9** Student case study: community and medical student partnership
>
> *An example of a partnership between medical students and a charity supporting young people with chronic illness or disabilities. https://www.thelunaproject.org.uk/Instagram-@thelunaprojectuk*
>
> The LUNA (Learning to Understand Needs and Abilities) Project is a small charity run by young people which started in 2018. The LUNA Project seeks to support young people with chronic illnesses, disabilities, and long-term health conditions. We also push for wider awareness because we believe that a world which *recognises* young people with disabilities is the first step in a world that works *for* young people and disabilities.
>
> Lots of our projects involve medical students, made easier by the number of medical students on the LUNA Committees who have both connections and are more aware of the gaps in medical education. For instance, our Science Communication Project was an interprofessional exercise where in groups, resources were created alongside people with lived experience. The resources focused on the science and Medicine behind certain conditions as we felt often this helped us to understand what was going on in our bodies a lot more but was often information not provided. We had over 80 students involved from across the UK and created some fantastic resources. We are also working alongside the medical school to create video interviews with some of our members about what it is like to live with a long-term health condition and "things they wish that doctors knew".
>
> It is hoped that these projects will encourage medical students – on placement, alongside lecture material, in their future careers and even in their everyday lives – to think about issues surrounding young people's health and the impact that both medical conditions and the encounters with medical professionals can have on a person.

involves a grasp of relevant social and ethical issues and challenges, yet these are often areas of the curriculum that are given little space (Collett et al., 2016).

It is important to consider what opportunities there are for students to engage with partners (including communities, policymakers, practitioners, and activists) within the curriculum. Partnership work is of benefit not only to the students, in grounding their understanding of the needs of particular communities, but also benefits the groups involved. An example of this is the partnership between LUNA, a charity supporting young people with chronic illness or disabilities, and medical students (Box 4.9). Community-based service-learning opportunities can be offered as electives, but it may be preferable to include required elements for all students (Faulkner et al., 2000).

> *As the concept of service learning becomes increasingly refined it behoves medical educators to include it as an essential part of the creation of 21st-century physicians. It moves the issue of professional development of altruism, humility and excellence beyond the realm of good intentions to measurable achievement (Woollard, 2006).*

Political engagement

While there is wide agreement that students and doctors have a responsibility to be aware of significant social and political issues such as health inequalities associated with climate change, the extent to which students should be engaged as political actors is perhaps more controversial and may vary in different countries. Brooks et al. (2020) suggested that

> *Political activity may constitute a key part of some students' identity if, for example, they are located in a country with a long history of student involvement in decision-making, at an institution that has provided their country with many politicians and/or on a course that requires engagement with social and political issues. For others, however, their understanding of what it means to be a student is likely to be substantially different.*

Medical schools should recognise that for some students, their civic professionalism will involve political engagement and activism. There are many ways in which both students and doctors are involved in work that is explicitly political. For example, Medact is an organisation committed to

> *Support health professionals from all disciplines to work together towards a world in which everyone can truly achieve and exercise their human right to health (https://www.medact.org).*

There is, however, the potential for disagreement over issues, and the school may be concerned about institutional reputation. As we noted above in relation to the use of social media, it should not be the intention of the school to "silence" its students. Professionalism is not a neutral category, and there is a risk that it is used to challenge student actions when those actions are intended to disrupt the status quo. There may well be times when student actions are rightly defined as unprofessional, but schools should be mindful of how and when such a label is applied in the context of civic professionalism. It is important to maintain an open dialogue, wherever possible to enable students' activism, and seek opportunities to adopt learning from students' experiences into the curriculum.

Conclusion

The student's role as a professional is important and contributes to the development of the student's professional identity. Professionalism is the way students conduct themselves in line with the expected behaviour. The student's role as a student doctor is a core aspect of professionalism, with the student expected to be a stellar example of what is expected of a doctor. Failure in this respect can prevent a student from continuing their studies.

As a professional learner, the student must take responsibility for their learning to achieve the expected goals. In doing so, the student must demonstrate integrity, honesty, and respect for teachers and colleagues.

The student as a professional must also work in partnership with the school to take responsibility for their health and well-being.

As a civic professional, the student has societal responsibilities that extend beyond their immediate roles as learners or student doctors that are increasingly recognised as core to being a medical professional.

The student should demonstrate professionalism in each of the roles described in this book, as a learning facilitator, an information provider, a curriculum developer, an assessor, a learner, a manager, and a scholar. Professionalism should be internalised by the student in the context of each of the roles. This works best when the student has a passion for and enjoyment in their work, and the medical school recognises their responsibility to provide a learning environment that supports all the dimensions of professionalism discussed in this chapter.

References

Baik, C., Larcombe, W., Brooker, A., 2019. How universities can enhance student mental wellbeing: The student perspective. High. Educ. Res. Dev. 38 (4), 674–687.

Barlow, C.J., Morrison, S., Stephens, H.O., Jenkins, E., Bailey, M.J., Pilcher, D., 2015. Unprofessional behaviour on social media by medical students. Med. J. Aust. 203 (11), 439.

BMA., 2020. Social Media as a Medical Student. https://www.bma.org.uk/advice-and-support/ethics/medical-students/ethics-toolkit-for-medical-students/social-media.

Brooks, R., Gupta, A., Jayadeva, S., Abrahams, J., Lažetić, P., 2020. Students as political actors? Similarities and differences across six European nations. Br. Educ. Res. J. 46 (6), 1193–1209.

Buckley, H., Steinert, Y., Regehr, G., Nimmon, L., 2019. When I say … community of practice. Med. Educ. 53, 763–765.

Chretien, K.C., Greysen, S.R., Chretien, J.P., Kind, T., 2009. Online posting of unprofessional content by medical students. JAMA. 302 (12), 1309–1315.

Close, L. 2019. 'Fun is the best way to learn': Lessons from Medsimscape- A Medical Simulation Escape Room Game. https://festivalofcreativelearning.wordpress.com/2019/08/08/fun-is-the-best-way-to-learn-lessons-from-medsimscape-a-medical-simulation-escape-room-game/.

Cochrane, E., Crook, E., 2021. STASHH: The next generation of genitourinary medicine doctors. Sex. Transm. Infect. 97, 323.

Collett, T., Brooks, L., Forrest, S., 2016. The history of sociology teaching in United Kingdom (UK) undergraduate medical education: an introduction and rallying call!. MedEdPublish. 5 (3).

Cruess, R.L., Cruess, S.R., Steinert, Y., 2018. Medicine as a community of practice: implications for medical education. Acad. Med. 93 (2), 185–191.

Daya, Z., Hearn, J.H., 2018. Mindfulness interventions in medical education: A systematic review of their impact on medical student stress, depression, fatigue and burnout. Med. Teach. 40 (2), 146–153.

Dyrbye, L.N., Massie, F.S., Eacker, A., et al., 2010. Relationship between burnout and professional conduct and attitudes among US medical students. JAMA. 304 (11), 1173–1180.

Dyrbye, L., Shanafelt, T., 2016. A narrative review on burnout experienced by medical students and residents. Med. Educ. 50 (1), 132–149.

Ellaway, R.H., Coral, J., Topps, D., Topps, M., 2015. Exploring digital professionalism. Med. Teach. 37 (9), 844–849.

Farrell, S.M., Kadhum, M., Lewis, T., Singh, G., Penzenstadler, L., Molodynski, A., 2019. Wellbeing and burnout amongst medical students in England. Int. Rev. Psychiatry. 31 (7-8), 579–583.

Faulkner, L.R., McCurdy, R.L., 2000. Teaching medical students social responsibility. Acad. Med. 75 (4), 346–350.

Gaufberg, E., Hafferty, F.W., 2021. The hidden curriculum. In: Dent, J.A., Harden, R.M., Hunt, D. (Eds.), A Practical Guide for Medical Teachers. Elsevier, London, UK.

General Medical Council and Medical Schools Council, 2021. Achieving Good Medical Practice: Guidance for Medical Students. https://www.gmc-uk.org/education/standards-guidance-and-curricula/guidance/student-professionalism-and-ftp/achieving-good-medical-practice.

Henning, M.A., Krägeloh, C.U., Dryer, R., Moir, F., Billington, R., Hill, A.G., 2018. Wellbeing in Higher Education: Cultivating a Healthy Lifestyle Among Faculty and Students. Routledge, Oxfordshire, UK.

Johnson, L., Malik, N., Gafson, I., Gostelow, N., Kavanagh, J., Griffin, A., Gishen, F., 2018. Improving patient safety by enhancing raising concerns at medical school. BMC. Med. Educ. 18, 171.

Kalter 2019. (https://www.aamc.org/news-insights/social-media-dilemma.

Koritz, A., Schadewald, P., 2015. Be the change: academics as civic professionals. Peer. Rev. 17 (3), 12–15.

Leedham-Green, K., Knight, A., Iedema, R., 2020. Developing professional identity in health professional students. In: Nestel, D., Reedy, G., McKenna, L., Gough, S. (Eds.), Clinical Education for the Health Professions. Springer, Singapore. pp. 1–21.

Lim, J.E.K., Selwyn, B.L., 2021. STASHH: Aims and foreseen benefits to medical students and pre-specialty trainees. Sex. Transm Infect. 97, 478.

McIntyre, K.R., Crawford, L.E., 2022. Outcomes for group working: Contextualising group work within professionalism frameworks. Med. Educ. 56 (5), 551.

O'Byrne, L., Gavin, B., Adamis, D., Lim, Y., McNicholas, F., 2021. Levels of stress in medical students due to COVID-19. J. Med. Ethics. 47, 383–388.

Orsmond, P., McMillan, H., Zvauya, R., 2022. It's how we practice that matters: Professional identity formation and legitimate peripheral participation in medical students: a qualitative study. BMC. Med. Educ. 22, 91.

O'Sullivan, H., van Mook, W., Fewtrell, R., Wass, V., 2012. Integrating professionalism into the curriculum: AMEE Guide No. 61. Med. Teach. 34 (2), e64–e77.

Pacheco, J.P., Giacomin, H.T., Tam, W.W., Ribeiro, T.B., Arab, C., Bezerra, I.M., Pinasco, G.C., 2017. Mental health problems among medical students in Brazil: A systematic review and meta-analysis. Braz. J. Psychiatry. 39 (4), 369–378.

Papadakis, M.A., Hodgson, C.S., Teherani, A., Kohatsu, N.D., 2004. Unprofessional behaviour in medical school is associated with subsequent disciplinary action by a state medical board. Acad. Med. 79 (3), 244–249.

Pronk, S.A., Gorter, S.L., van Luijk, S.J., et al., 2021. Perception of social media behaviour among medical students, residents and medical specialists. Perspect. Med. Educ. 10, 215–221.

Ranmuthugala, G., Plumb, J.J., Cunningham, F.C., Georgiou, A., Westbrook, J.I., Braithwaite, J, 2011. How and why are communities of practice established in the healthcare sector? A systematic review of the literature. BMC Health Serv. Res. 11, 273.

Sarraf-Yazdi, S., Teo, N., How, A.E.H., et al., 2021. A Scoping Review of Professional Identity Formation in Undergraduate Medical Education. J. Gen. Intern. Med. 36, 3511–3521.

Sattar, K., Akram, A., Ahmad, T., Bashir, U., 2021. Professionalism development of undergraduate medical students: Effect of time and transition. Medicine. 100 (9), e23580.

Saunders, P.A., Tractenberg, R.E., Chaterji, R., Amri, H., Harazduk, N., Gordon, J.S., Lumpkin, M., Haramati, A., 2007. Promoting self-awareness and reflection through an experiential Mind-Body Skills course for first year medical students. Med. Teach. 29 (8), 778–784.

Scherer, L.A., Leshner, A.I., 2021. Mental Health, Substance Use, and Wellbeing in Higher Education: Supporting the Whole Student. National Academies Press, Washington, D.C., USA.

Slavin, S., 2019. MEd reflections on a decade leading a medical student well-being initiative. Academic Medicine. 94 (6), 771–774.

Staffaroni, A., Rush, C.L., Graves, K.D., Hendrix, K., Haramati, A., Harazduk, N., 2017. Long-term follow-up of mind-body medicine practices among medical school graduates. Med. Teach. 39 (12), 1275–1283.

Sullivan, W.H., Benner, P., 2005. Challenges to professionalism: Work integrity and the call to renew and strengthen the social contract of the professions. Am. J. Crit. Care. 14 (1), 78–80, 84.

UNESCO International Institute for Higher Education in Latin America and the Caribbean. 2021. Thinking Higher and Beyond: Perspectives and Futures of Higher Education in 2050. Accessed online 14/06/2022 at https://unesdoc.unesco.org/ark:/48223/pf0000377530.

Vanderbilt Medical School. Vanderbilt School of Medicine Catalog. Vanderbilt University, accessed on 25/03/2022 at https://www.vumc.org/faculty/sites/vumc.org.faculty/files/public_files/compact4teachers_learners05.pdf.

Wilkes, C., Lewis, T., Brager, N., Bulloch, A., MacMaster, F., Paget, M., Holm, J., Farrell, S.M., Ventriglio, A., 2019. Wellbeing and mental health amongst medical students in Canada. Int. Rev. Psychiatry. 31 (7–8), 584–587.

Woollard, R.F., 2006. Caring for a common future: Medical schools' social accountability. Med. Educ. 40, 301–313.

York, M., Langford, K., Davidson, M., Hemingway, C., Russell, R., Neeley, M., Fleming, A., 2021. Becoming active bystanders and advocates: teaching medical students to respond to bias in the clinical setting. MedEdPORTAL. 17, 11175.

The student as a facilitator of their own learning   5

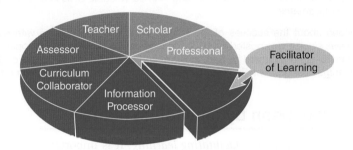

Facilitating learning

Learning is a student's priority and, consistent with the theme of student engagement, the role of students in facilitating their own learning is attracting increasing recognition.

Traditionally, the facilitation of learning was seen as the responsibility of the teacher (Harden and Lilley, 2018), with the teacher transmitting knowledge and unlocking in the student their potential to learn. Student-facilitated learning represents a shift in the power relationship between teacher and student and has to be a shared teacher-student function. One result of the COVID-19 pandemic educationally has been a move to a greater emphasis on remote or online learning and on digital learning environments. Students have had to assume a greater measure of responsibility for managing and facilitating their own learning with less guidance or direction received from the teacher.

The power of students facilitating their own learning was demonstrated in 2010 in a school in Massachusetts, USA. In *The Independent Project*, as described in Box 5.1, students successfully designed and ran their own school programme for a semester (Wehmeyer and Zhao, 2020). The facilitation of their learning by the student was demonstrated to be a very real and possible task.

In this chapter, we discuss the two core concepts – learning and facilitation. We then consider approaches to understanding student-facilitated learning and consider some tools that support and guide students in this role.

Box 5.1 Students run their own school

In *The Independent Project* in Massachusetts, USA, students owned and facilitated their own learning for one semester by developing and managing their own curriculum (Wehmeyer and Zhao, 2020). Although students sought advice from teachers, they followed their own curriculum without taking other classes. They were responsible for their own learning, monitoring each other's work and providing feedback to one another. Despite some pushback from faculty and parents, the school's Curriculum Steering Committee and the Board approved the proposed programme, and the experiment began in 2010.

The project proved to be a huge success. The results were transformative with students who had struggled in the conventional classroom flourishing in their own school. Students produced substantial and authentic work and learned valuable skills in time management and helping classmates.

A short video about the success of the project went viral on YouTube with more than 200,000 views since it was posted in 2013. The project was also the central topic of a book published in 2016, co-authored by Samuel Levin and Susan Engel – *A School of Our Own: The Story of the First Student-Run High School and a New Vision for American Education*.

What do we mean by facilitating learning?

The theme of this chapter is *facilitating learning*. It is important to address what we understand as learning. In his book *"And What Do You Mean by Learning?"* Seymour B. Sarason (2004) notes that while "learning" is at or near the top of the most frequently used words in education literature, its meaning is not always explicitly addressed. Ambrose et al. (2010, p. 3) define learning as

"A process that leads to change, which occurs as a result of experience and increases the potential for improved performance and future learning"

They highlight three key aspects of this definition:

1. Learning is a process, not a product. However, because this process takes place in the mind, we can only infer that it has occurred from students' products or performances.

2. Learning involves change in knowledge, beliefs, behaviors, or attitudes. This change unfolds over time; it is not fleeting but rather has a lasting impact on how students think and act.

3. Learning is not something done to students, but rather something students themselves do. It is the direct result of how students interpret and respond to their experiences — conscious and unconscious, past and present.

By facilitation, we mean the actions and processes involved in helping learning happen and increasing the likelihood of it happening effectively. There are many aspects of facilitating learning that involve actions by faculty and the medical school. Doug Belshaw (2016) captured, in his blog, the concept of facilitation from a teacher's perspective, with the analogy of a teacher standing with their students on one side of a river and helping them across to the other side using stepping stones. In this metaphor, the teacher may not be able to remove the obstruction (the river) but can help the student to cross (they may have not been able to do so alone) or make it easier (they may have been able to wade across, but the stones make crossing easier). Facilitating may mean creating different modes of crossing or allowing students to cross the river at earlier/later points.

Returning to the definition of learning above, "learning is not done to students, but rather something students themselves do". In the facilitator role, it is the student rather than the teacher who finds potential stepping stones to cross the river, find an alternative crossing, or make it easier by tailoring their learning. The student may raise the question of why it is necessary to cross the river at all.

The student as a self-directed learner

The traditional approach to learning in medical education assumes that students need to be made aware of what they should be learning, but that control for planning the learning programme should rest with teachers, not students. We need to go beyond the idea that education is something that is provided for students and accept the concept that education is something that students can create for themselves. Students have the capacity to facilitate their own learning and make choices as to what, how, where, when, and with whom they should be learning.

This is the locus for the concept of the student as a self-directed learner. In self-directed learning, the learner takes control over and is responsible for their own learning. The student takes the initiative (Knowles, 1975) in:

- Diagnosing their learning needs – identifying what they should learn
- Formulating goals for their learning
- Identifying opportunities to help them achieve their goals
- Choosing and implementing appropriate learning strategies
- Evaluating their learning outcomes

The self-directed learner decides what needs to be learned and how this learning is best accomplished. This entails considering their schedule for work and developing a sustainable routine, for example, how many hours in the day and when (Mittal et al. 2021).

In medical education, there is a continuing search from a teacher's perspective for the most effective educational approach or strategy involving, for example, the use of technology or a restructuring of the curriculum. It may, however, be more productive, as ten Cate et al. (2010) suggests, to explore further how students can be better engaged as learners.

ten Cate et al. describe self-determination theory (SDT) and its application to learning in AMEE Guide 59 (2011). They suggest that traditionally

> *Many teachers and institutions think that they are most successful if they control most of student activities based on a carefully designed curriculum and*

well-chosen teaching methods. However, SDT informs us that by not allowing students to choose how to learn for themselves, they are less likely to identify with the material or to integrate it and thus will be less likely to remember what they have learned and what they do retain will be less integrated into their identity as developing physicians.

Self-determined learning theory encompasses three needs that are key to the psychology of motivational processes (Ryan and Deci, 2000):

- *The need for autonomy:* the individual can choose what they want to do. They fully endorse and concur with the behaviour they are engaged in. Some of the characteristics of autonomy-supportive teaching were described by Wehmeyer and Zhow (Box 5.2)
- *The need for competence:* the desire to feel confident and effective or competent in whatever actions are pursued
- *The need for relatedness:* the desire to feel connected with others and a sense of belongingness

However, it is important to place in context the internal psychological factors that shape self-directed learning. Consideration should also be given to the external learning environment and the ways in which that can support or hinder students' self-directed learning needs.

Appropriate learning environments can be arranged where students play a role in facilitating their own learning, and where self-directed learning harnesses the power of student autonomy and student ownership to motivate students. For example, in PBL, where there is evidence of student engagement, ten Cate (2011) suggests that the increase found in student motivation is in concordance with the increased self-determination of students to meet the three psychological needs described above. Students feel more autonomous as they formulate their own learning objectives. Relatedness is stimulated as groups of students work together, and there is a satisfactory feeling of competence when students explain mastered content to their peers.

Box 5.2 The characteristics of autonomy-supportive teaching as described by Wehmeyer and Zhao (p. 35)

- Recognising students' strengths and abilities rather than limitations
- Promoting students' volitional actions and perceptions of choice rather than dependency and pressure
- Harnessing the power of students' passions and curiosity rather than conformity and standardisation
- Facilitating students' agency and ownership over learning rather than compliance and obedience

---

Clinical learning environments offer students opportunities for self-directed learning. A degree of responsibility for patients may increase a sense of autonomy and develop clinical competence, and a feeling of relatedness can be fostered as members of a clinical team. However, there may be challenges for students in making the transition from pre-clinical to clinical learning environments. An expectation of self-directed learning is not always accompanied by necessary support, given the other demands on educators' time in a clinical context (Cho et al., 2017). For example, there may be a greater expectation that students define the task, by setting their own learning objectives. This may be new to some students, and they may need guidance in taking on this responsibility for their learning.

The scope and manner of students' roles as self-directed learners are also shaped by the wider values and practices of student engagement. For example, in *The Independent Project* described in Box 5.1, students had a leading role in defining the learning task; they took responsibility for developing and implementing their curriculum over a semester. This highlights the potential for applying the concept of self-directed learning at a more macro level, to encourage student self-determination; not only for the micro tasks involved in their learning, but for the curriculum itself. We explore this further in Chapter 7.

While all students will engage to varying extents and in different ways, as self-directed learners, some may face specific challenges. There is clear evidence of inequity in students' attainment and experiences that are important to consider in the context of the self-determined learner. Students' perception of competence may be shaped by their background, experiences and identity; those coming from non-traditional backgrounds may feel less confident in their academic ability. Coming from a different background to those around them may also impact their need to relate. Students from widening participation backgrounds can often feel like outsiders, and this lack of belonging has been highlighted as significant for understanding the differential attainment of students from minoritised groups (Krstić et al., 2021). It is likely that this also has an impact on their potential to become self-determined learners.

Self-Regulated learning

Sometimes used interchangeably with "self-directed learning" is the term "self-regulated learning" without a clear distinction being made between the two terms (Gandomkar and Sandars, 2018; Cleary and Sandars, 2011). The two terms have similarities. Both describe active participation by the learner in setting goals and choices in the implementation of appropriate learning strategies. Differences, however, have been recognised between the two terms. The self-directed learner may be viewed as a macro or broader concept that encompasses self-regulated learning. Self-regulated learning is

A cyclical learning process to plan, self-monitor and dynamically adapt motivation and learning strategies to ensure effective learning (Sandars and Walsh, 2021).

As noted by Gandomkar and Sandars (2018)

An effective self-directed learner must be an effective self-regulated learner, using a variety of key SRL processes to achieve their self-identified chosen

goals (Brydges et al. 2010). However, an effective self-regulated learner is frequently not a self-directed learner, with learning goals being externally formulated by their teacher.

Education principles embedded in student-facilitated learning

Four education features (the FAIR principles) that facilitate students' learning are Feedback, Activity, Individualisation, and Relevance (Harden and Laidlaw, 2021).

Feedback

Feedback about their performance and achievement of the learning outcomes makes an important contribution to the student's actions as a self-directed learner. Appropriate feedback about their performance should influence their next choice of educational strategies and learning resources and their further learning.

Much of the work relating to feedback has concerned how the teacher communicates to the student about gaps or deficiencies relating to their performance, as well as reinforcing good performance. Feedback, however, is also a two-way communication between the teacher and learner with discussions about the student's improvements in practice and about the personal growth of the student. The student should know how to ask for appropriate feedback when this is not provided.

Activity

A feature of self-directed learning (and self-regulated learning) is that the student actively participates in facilitating their learning. The student is not simply a receptacle to be filled with the necessary knowledge, skills, and attitude but is a partner who should be actively engaged in the process.

> *Learning is not a spectator sport. Students do not learn much by sitting in classes listening to teachers memorising pre-packaged assignments and spitting out answers. They must talk about what they are learning, write about it, relate it to past experiences, and apply it to their daily life (Chickering and Gamson, 1991).*

In Chapter 6 we consider further how a student can adopt an active approach to their learning.

Individualisation

Students have different learning needs and learn in different ways. With the student engaged as a partner in the learning process, the education programme should adapt to these needs. As self-directed learners, the students should take responsibility by reflecting on their own learning and seeking resources that best address their needs. This may involve engaging in what has been described as a "parallel curriculum", the spaces where students learn, often from each other, and in ways over which they have choice and control (Quirk and Chumley, 2018).

Relevance

The fourth component of the FAIR model is relevance. To assist the student as a self-directed learner in deciding what they should learn, they need to recognise the relevance of their studies to their future work as a doctor. This is critical for effective learning and the maintenance of the learner's interests and motivation. Relevance is encouraged, for example, in a vertically integrated curriculum with clinical experiences available in the early years and learning structured around clinical problems or presentations. Much of the responsibility for ensuring relevance sits with the teachers and programme teams. However, students can also adopt self-learning approaches that apply similar principles; for example, by creating their own clinical scenarios to test the application of their knowledge.

A further aspect of relevance relates to the importance of ensuring that the curriculum reflects the students and the wider communities they will serve as doctors. Core to this is the development of relevant curricula that actively and intentionally engage with discrimination; often discussed as the need to "decolonise", "liberate", or make the curriculum more "inclusive". Students can support this work by highlighting examples of good/bad practice, though the burden that engaging in activism/advocacy can have on students should be kept in mind and support should be in place for students who partake in this work.

Inclusivity

We can add another principle to the FAIR model - Inclusivity. Approaches to equality, diversity and inclusion in medical education are shifting from interventions responding to the needs of individual or specific groups of students, to systemic change that "anticipates and plans for entitlements of the evolving student population" (Morgan and Houghton, 2011). Learning contexts should be developed, within which not just some but all students feel supported to facilitate their own learning. It is important to ensure that teacher and student expectations related to self-determined learning do not reinforce inequities and that any systemic issues that can pose challenges to the adoption of the self-directed learning role are addressed. For example, students with caring responsibilities may have less time available to be able to engage in the process of determining their own learning. They may also be disadvantaged by organisational issues: for example in some medical schools, placement timetables are often released to students very close to the start of the placement making it more challenging for those with other work or caring responsibilities to organise their lives to support their role as self-determined learners. Moreover, discrimination may result in reduced learning opportunities. Students have reported examples of clinical teachers favouring male students in question rounds and offering men additional learning opportunities. One study reported that ethnic minority students found cultural issues to be a barrier to participation in clinical skills; for example, a student who stopped wearing their hijab, as they found it reduced their chance of being selected to participate (Vaughan 2013). Such experiences may limit students' potential to be self-determined learners and demonstrate the need for an inclusive approach.

Tools to facilitate learning

A range of tools, notably study guides, curriculum maps, and statements of learning outcomes, can be used to facilitate learning (Figure 5.1). Their use by the teacher is described in the Eight Roles of the Medical Teacher (Harden and Lilley, 2018). The same tools, however, can be used by the student to facilitate their own learning.

Study guides

A study guide is a powerful tool that can be employed by students to facilitate their learning. A study guide in paper or electronic form provides the student with advice as to what they should be learning at a given point in time. Advice may be given as to the optimum selection of learning experiences to match the student's personal needs and the opportunities provided to allow the student to assess their achievement of the learning outcomes. The guide may also include practical hints as to how students can tackle potential difficulties and problems that may arise in the course of their studies. The use of study guides to facilitate learning is described in AMEE Guide 16 (Harden et al., 1999a).

The study guide can be seen as the equivalent for the individual traveller of the advice given by the tour agency as to how the traveller can have a safe journey and get the maximum benefit from the trip.

A curriculum map

A curriculum map is a visual representation of a curriculum that shows how the different elements, including the expected learning outcomes, the teaching and

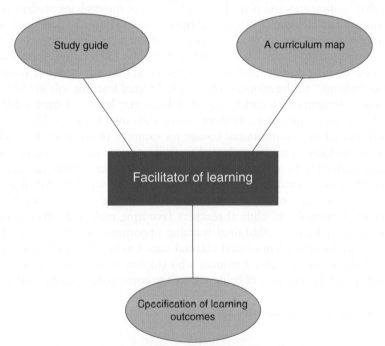

Figure 5.1 Tools for the self-directed learner to facilitate their learning.

learning opportunities, and the assessment, relate to one another (Harden, 2011) Figure 5.2. Imagine the student as a traveller to a distant land. The map will illustrate the different desired destinations (equivalent to the learning outcomes in a curriculum map) and how the destinations can be accessed by road, rail, or air (equivalent in the curriculum map to the available learning opportunities and resources). In the same way that a traveller finds a map of their journey helpful, the student will find that a map of their curriculum facilitates their education journey.

The map can be explored using different lenses. For example, the student can explore the expected learning outcomes relating to the *communication skills* outcome domain and can identify how these are addressed in different courses in the curriculum, along with the learning opportunities available to support their learning, such as a simulated patient encounter in a clinical skills laboratory. Alternatively, the map can be explored with a focus on *courses or modules*, for example, the cardiovascular system module, with the details of the expected learning outcomes, information about the lectures and other resources available highlighted. The student can identify available learning opportunities on the curriculum map in relation to each of the specified learning outcomes and how each outcome is reflected in the assessment.

In Figure 5.2, the learning outcomes are shown in relation to each body system including, for example, mastery of specified clinical skills. One of the skills identified is blood pressure measurement. Each of the nodes on the map, for example, blood pressure measurement, is related to the available learning opportunities, in the case of BP measurement studying a video of the procedure, experiencing the technique in the simulation laboratory or in the clinical setting. Also identified is how the procedure is assessed, for example, in an OSCE, a tutor's report or from the student's portfolio. In the list of clinical presentations addressed in the curriculum the appropriate presentation is displayed – hypertension.

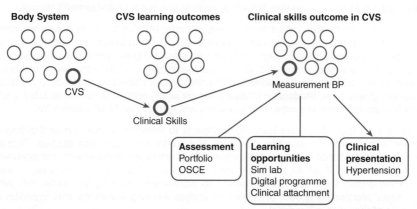

Figure 5.2 A curriculum map showing measurement of blood pressure (BP) as a required clinical skill in the cardiovascular system (CVS). Clinical presentation, learning opportunities and assessment are identified (Harden and Laidlaw 2021). Source: Modified from Ronald Harden, Jennifer Laidlaw. *Essential Skills for a Medical Teacher, 3e*, Mapping the curriculum, Figure 17.1, Edinburgh, Elsevier LTD, 2021.

Learning outcomes

Perhaps one of the most important developments in medical education in the past two decades has been the move to an outcome-based education (OBE) approach, with the expected learning outcomes matched with the teaching and learning methods offered, and the assessment (Harden et al., 1999b).

A significant advantage of an OBE approach is that it offers the student the autonomy to take responsibility for their own learning and to select appropriate teaching and learning methods matched to the expected learning outcomes. The availability of the set of learning outcomes empowers the student to facilitate their own learning programme. Lack of information about the learning outcomes expected on completion of a course is the equivalent of engaging in a "magical mystery tour", where the destination is unknown. If a student is aware of where they should be going as illustrated on the curriculum map and the learning outcomes to be achieved, they can decide how to best achieve these outcomes by identifying the most appropriate learning strategies and use of resources for that specific student. They can also evaluate their progress in reaching the target of the exit learning outcomes. Empowering students in this way can be challenging for teachers, as students may decide that the teaching methods provided do not best meet their needs; for example, they may feel that attending the lectures is not required to facilitate their achieving the learning outcomes.

A student case study in Box 5.3 highlights the challenges that neurodivergent students may experience in becoming self-directed learners and the importance of access to the right tools, including learning outcomes, to support their learning.

Box 5.3 Student case study - not fitting the "one size fits all"

Reflections on the challenges for a neurodivergent student and the steps taken to facilitate her own learning, by Catriona McVey, University of Manchester

As a medical student with a specific learning difficulty, I am all too aware that medical education often has a "one size fits all" approach to educating tomorrow's doctors.

My diagnosis of attention deficit hyperactivity disorder (ADHD) came as a surprise, more than halfway through my second year at medical school. I had long believed that I was not intelligent, or not trying hard enough, and that was why I had barely passed my exams so far. I told my medical school about my diagnosis, but there wasn't any additional learning support available beyond the study skills workshops I'd already attended numerous times, on account of being a dropout risk. Students with disabilities are legally entitled to accommodations, so I quickly arranged things like extra time for exams and a specialised study skills tutor.

I changed my focus from rote-learning flashcards to achieving a deep understanding of content with flowcharts, practice questions and working through case studies. Despite being told by staff that lecture recordings were not adequate replacements for attending in person, I found it easier to concentrate on lectures when I did so from home with the video slightly sped up. I have learned to advocate for myself, as I know that with my slower processing speed, the ability to access learning outcomes and materials in advance of the class is essential.

When I received my first set of exam results after my diagnosis of ADHD, I had a serious concern that the university would suspect me of cheating. I had scored just 1% below a first class after previously only ever reaching the dizzy heights of 4% above the pass mark – barely even a third class. Since then, I have continued to improve academically and finally feel like I belong in medical school.

Where a study guide, a curriculum map, and a set of learning outcomes are not available, students can work together to bring pressure on the school to fill the gap and can work with teachers and programme managers to remedy the deficiency. We come back to this in Chapters 7 and 11.

Peer learning

The sections above have focused mainly on students as individual learners. Students can also facilitate their learning by learning together with another student(s) – peer learning. Some of this will happen during class time but can also form part of their self-study or class preparation time. Two forms of peer learning – cooperative and collaborative – have been described (Box 5.4).

Cooperative learning

Students learn with their peers in a group, working together on a joint task, with each student having the same status. The teacher often acts as an organiser or facilitator of the group task. A jigsaw approach is one of the most well-known types of cooperative learning with each member becoming an expert in one part of the topic so that the whole picture can be completed.

> *Cooperative learning is viewed as requiring division of labour among participants, with each member being responsible for sub-tasks being resolved individually and then the group assembling the different portions into the group task (Topping et al., 2017, p. 3).*

Problem-based learning can be viewed as an example of cooperative learning; the students work together in groups to tackle a problem. As a group, they need to identify what is necessary to know in order to answer the problem. Work is then shared by students in the group with students coming together to share their knowledge with a view to answering the problem.

Some common components that define cooperative learning are (Buchs, 2016):

- *Positive goal interdependence:* Group members perceive that they achieve a common educational goal and that the input of each of them allows achievement of the goal. It is not just one person doing all of the work.
- *Personal responsibility and group accountability:* Learners feel responsible for their own learning and for helping others to learn in the group.

Box 5.4   An example of peer collaboration

Students worked in pairs to study online a programme addressing the cardiovascular system (Khogali et al., 2011)

Students studying the integrated Dundee cardiovascular system programme use an online learning resource to facilitate their learning. Some students chose to study this in pairs rather than work through it on their own or in a larger group. The students in the pair assisted each other in learning the subject and answering questions raised during the programme, discussing their answers, and helping each other when aspects of the programme were not clear.

- *Teachers structure the group work:* To encourage peer interactions and cooperation in the group the teacher guides and facilitates the interactive process and ensures that the group have specific goals, tasks, and resources.

The climate of the traditional curriculum may encourage competition between students rather than cooperation. Students may need a cooperative nudge with an explanation as to why and how they should cooperate. The preparation of students to cooperate increases the likelihood of success in cooperative learning.

Collaborative learning

Peer collaboration is an approach to peer learning where two or more students facilitate their learning by learning together with none assuming a dominant pedagogical role. Peer collaboration represents a more student-centred approach compared to cooperative learning where the teacher has an important role in managing the group's activities; it is assumed that the students have the motivation and skills to manage their own learning together. Smith and McGregor (1992) as cited by Davidson and Major (2014) described the essential features of collaborative learning

> In most collaborative learning situations students are working in groups of two or more, mutually searching for understanding, solutions, or meaning, or creating a product. There is a wide variability in collaborative learning activities but most centre on the student's exploration or application of the course material.

An example of peer collaboration in which students chose to study together in pairs is given in Box 5.4.

In Box 5.5, we present a student case study that beautifully illustrates the potential for collaborative, self-determined learning through the sharing of poetry to reflect on the experience of dissection.

Challenges of peer learning

Cooperative and collaborative learning can be valuable approaches to supporting students' self-determined learning but can be challenging for some students. Students have reported concerns about the learning impact when some group members dominate or negatively criticise the contributions of peers (Iqbal et al., 2016). This may be seen as part of students' learning how to work collaboratively as part of a team, essential to medical practice. However, some groups may be disproportionately impacted by such experiences. As we noted above, students from minoritised groups may feel "other" and so may feel less confident when participating in group activities. Students also report microaggressions in their interactions with other students, which may also have a negative impact on their learning experience. While cooperative learning that is embedded in the curriculum can be monitored by facilitators, more informal, student-organised forms of collaborative learning may be more difficult to manage. It is important to provide advice to students on what collaborative learning can offer, but also on the potential challenges and how

Box 5.5   Student case study: Collaborative learning through poetry

A reflection on writing poetry to facilitate learning, by Rumaisa Zubairi, University of Glasgow

The subtle shifting that takes place in the medical student as they transition from (typically) a regular teenager to a doctor witnessing the momentous occasions of the entrance of life and death is remarkable. In hospital, we witness some of the most profound moments in our patients' lives as they are brought to tears by pain or disclose the trauma of a difficult childhood for the first time. While formal medical school teaching hurls classification criteria and management protocols for what seems like an endless list of ailments, students are perhaps less well prepared to deal with what happens when the treatments must stop and the Great Inevitable happens. Unsure how to respond, not yet having had the time to completely absorb the cryptic lessons of "informal learning", the student can feel overwhelmed and a little bit useless.

At such a time, we should debrief with an understanding member of the team. But they will not be there when our mind is mulling over the day's events later on. This turning inward is only natural, and I feel we might as well try to make the most of it by channelling our reflections into a creative medium. I was greatly moved by my first experience of the dissection hall and wrote a poem about it, which I shared it with my peers. Hearing it gave many of them permission to acknowledge and voice their own unshared feelings. We realised that the experience had left its mark on all of us, despite our efforts to hide the fact. I again shared a poem I wrote at the end of my first placement with those who were on the block with me. Our conversation shifted to the lessons we learned during the block: not science and drugs, but about the mental toll of working with the ill.

Writing these pieces allowed me to reveal layers of meaning within those interactions and take ownership of them, and sharing them allowed us to come to a communal understanding, broach unspoken territories, and acknowledge how far we had come. My poems gave a form to murky unknowns, and we realised that by learning in a way that transcends textbooks, that the compassion and reflection that draws us to these poems is precisely what will allow us to handle those difficult and uncertain moments with empathy and wisdom.

to address them. Clear lines of reporting any concerns should also be made available to students, whether the learning is within the curriculum or takes place more informally. There may also be a barrier to some students engaging in informal peer learning; those with other time-consuming responsibilities may have less time or may find it more difficult to arrange peer meetings. Schools should ensure that sufficient time is given for formal peer learning activities and that advice is offered regarding the timing of informal peer learning.

The student as a facilitator of their own learning in relation to their other roles

Each of the student's roles can contribute in different ways to the facilitation of learning by the student. The extent and ways in which a student will facilitate their learning via these roles will vary depending on the institutional, cultural, and individual context in which they are studying.

The student as an information processor and information seeker (Chapter 6)

The student can facilitate their learning through a better understanding and adoption of a range of strategies for processing the information they receive in lectures, texts, small group work, and clinical experiences; and for seeking information relevant to their learning.

The student as a curriculum collaborator and evaluator (Chapter 7)

The student's engagement with the curriculum, as a collaborator, can facilitate their learning. As noted by Ambrose et al. (2017)

> *The more that students can be involved in the creation of the design of the curriculum and engaged in the quality improvements of the courses and the teaching, the more the student gains the sense of ownership for their own learning.*

The student as an assessor (Chapter 8)

The move from assessment-of-learning to assessment-for-learning recognises that assessment has a key role to play in facilitating learning. Encouraging self-assessment as part of learning, teaching, and assessment can help students to become self-determined learners.

The student as a teacher (Chapter 9)

The student can facilitate their learning of a subject by teaching it. The increasing adoption of peer teaching benefits not only the tutee but also the student as the tutor.

The student as a scholar (Chapter 10)

Through engagement in the wider scholarship of teaching and research, students can develop and deepen skills that may enhance their learning in the programme.

The student as a professional (Chapter 11)

The student is expected to adopt a professional approach to their studies and exhibit professionalism not only as a student doctor but also as a learner with regard to their learning-related behaviour and relationship with colleagues and teachers. Part of this professionalism is their development as self-directed learners.

Conclusion

Not in question is that making learning achievable, accessible, enjoyable, and effective is a key responsibility of the teacher and that medical schools have a core part to play in ensuring that the educational approach, systems, and structures of learning support students. The student, however, also has an important responsibility to facilitate their own learning.

As self-determined learners, students regulate their own learning by making use of tools such as study guides, curriculum maps, and statements of expected learning outcomes. In facilitating their learning, they can work individually or collaboratively with peers. The student's role as a facilitator of learning is embedded in all seven roles for the student described in the subsequent chapters of this text.

References

Ambrose, S.A., Bridges, M.W., DiPietro, M., Lovett, M.C., Norman, M.K., 2010. How learning works: Seven research-based principles for smart teaching. Jossey-Bass, San Francisco, California, USA.

Ambrose, S.A., Waechter, D.M., Hunt, D., 2017. Student engagement in learning 2017. In: Dent, J.A., Harden, R.M., Hunt, D. (Eds.), A Practical Guide for Medical Teachers. Elsevier, London, UK.

Belshaw, D., 2016. How to use metaphors to generate badge-based pathways. http://dougbelshaw.com/blog/2016/06/28/badge-pathway-metaphors.

Brydges, R., Dubrowski, A., Regehr, G., 2010. A new concept of unsupervised learning: Directed self-guided learning in the health professions. Acad. Med. 85, S49–S55.

Buchs, C., Gilles, I., Antonietti, J.P., Butera, F., 2016. Why students need to be prepared to cooperate: A cooperative nudge in statistics learning at university. Educ. Psych. 36 (5), 956–974.

Chickering, A.W., Gamson, Z.F., 1991. Seven principles of good practice in undergraduate education. New Direct Teach. Learn. 47, 63–69.

Cho, K.K., Marjadi, B., Langendyk, V., Hu, W., 2017. The self-regulated learning of medical students in the clinical environment – a scoping review. BMC Med. Educ. 17 (112).

Cleary, T.J., Sandars, J., 2011. Assessing self-regulatory processes during clinical skill performance: A pilot study. Med. Teach. 33 (7), e368–e374.

Davidson, N., Major, C.H., 2014. Boundary crossings: cooperative learning, collaborative learning, and problem-based learning. J. Excel. Coll. Teach. 25 (3-4), 7–55.

Gandomkar, R., Sandars, J., 2018. Clearing the confusion about self-directed learning and self-regulated learning. Med. Teach. 40 (8), 862–863.

Harden, R.M., Laidlaw, J.M., Hesketh, E.A., 1999a. AMEE Medical Education Guide No 16: Study guides-their use and preparation. Med. Teach. 21 (3), 248–265.

Harden, R.M., Crosby, J.R., Davis, M.H., 1999b. AMEE Guide No. 14: Outcome-based education: Part 1-An introduction to outcome-based education. Med. Teach. 21 (1), 7–14.

Harden, R.M., Laidlaw, J.M., 2021. Essential Skills for a Medical Teacher (3rd ed). Elsevier, London, UK.

Harden, R.M., Lilley, P.M., 2018. The Eight Roles of the Medical Teacher. Elsevier, London, UK.

Iqbal, M., Velan, G.M., O'Sullivan, A.J., Balasooriya, C, 2016. Differential impact of student behaviours on group interaction and collaborative learning: Medical students' and tutors' perspectives. BMC Med. Educ. 16, 217.

Khogali, S., Davies, D.A., Donnan, P.T., Gray, A., Harden, R.M., McDonald, J., Pippard, M.J., Pringle, S.D., Yu, N., 2011. Integration of e-learning resources into a medical school curriculum. Med. Teach. 33 (4), 311–318.

Knowles, M.S., 1975. Self-Directed Learning: A Guide for Learners and Teachers. Association Press, New York, New York, USA.

Krstić, C., Krstić, L., Tulloch, A., Agius, S., Warren, A., Doody, G.A., 2021. The experience of widening participation students in undergraduate medical education in the UK: A qualitative systematic review. Med. Teach. 43 (9), 1044–1053.

Levin, S., Engel, S.L., 2016. A School of Our Own. New Press, New York, New York, USA.

Mittal, S., Lau, V., Prior, K., Ewer, J. 2021. Twelve tips for medical students on how to maximise remote learning. Med Teach. Epub ahead of print. https://doi.org/10.1080/0142159X.2021.1912308.

Morgan, H., Houghton, A. 2011. Inclusive curriculum design in higher education. Considerations for effective practice across and within subject areas. https://www.advance-he.ac.uk/knowledge-hub/inclusive-curriculum-design-higher-education.

Quirk, M., Chumley, H., 2018. The adaptive medical curriculum: A model for continuous improvement. Med. Teach. 40 (8), 786–790.

Ryan, R.M., Deci, E.L., 2000. Self-determination theory and the facilitation of intrinsic motivation, social development, and well-being. Am. Psychol. 55 (1), 68–78.

Sandars, J., Cleary, T.J., 2011. Self-regulation theory: Applications to medical education: AMEE Guide No. 58. Med. Teach. 33 (11), 875–886.

Sandars, J., Walsh, K., 2021. Independent Learning and Distance Learning. In: Dent, J., Harden, R.M., Hunt, D. (Eds.), A Practical Guide for Medical Teachers. Elsevier, London, UK.

Sarason, S.B., 2004. And what do you mean by learning? Heinemann, Portsmouth, New Hampshire, USA.

ten Cate, T.J., Kusurkar, R.A., Williams, G.C., 2011. How self-determination theory can assist our understanding of the teaching and learning processes in medical education. AMEE guide No. 59. Med. Teach. 33 (12), 961–973.

Topping, K., Buchs, C., Duran, D., & Van Keer, H., 2017. Effective peer learning: From principles to practical implementation. Taylor & Francis.

Vaughan, S., 2013. Medical students' experience and achievement: The effect of ethnicity and social networks (PhD thesis). University of Manchester, Manchester, UK. Accessed on 20/06/22 at https://www.research.manchester.ac.uk/portal/en/theses/medical-students-experience-and-achievement-the-effect-of-ethnicity-and-social-networks(bbde8916-2914-44c8-a340-2b4c0c0b56a4).html.

Wehmeyer, M., Zhao, Y., 2020. Teaching Students to Become Self-Directed Learners. ASCD, Alexandria, Virginia, USA.

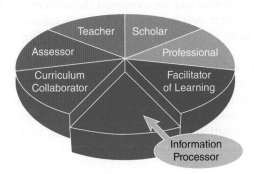

The student as a learner and an information processor

A doctor uses information gained in medical school to inform their work as a medical practitioner and to support their clinical decisions relating to a patient's potential diagnosis, appropriate investigations, and individual management plans. Acquiring and processing the necessary information is a key role for the student. The role of information processor, it can be argued, is perhaps the most traditional student role we describe.

Traditionally teachers were seen as dispensers of information, as described by Harden and Lilley (2018) with students as processors of this information. While ensuring that the student, on graduation, has the necessary knowledge base is the responsibility of the medical school, as described in Chapter 1, the move from teacher-centred to student-centred learning shifts some responsibility for information processing and seeking from the teacher to the student. This student's role as information processor has gained importance and is changing in the new economy of information.

- The *quantity of information* to be processed by the student has increased exponentially with the rapid expansion of knowledge in medicine and the biomedical sciences, and with the development of new areas of study such as patient safety and clinical reasoning. It is estimated that there are over 6000 scientific papers published each day (Gibney, 2014).

- The *developments in information technologies* and the increasing complexity of information technology as a science requires greater information literacy on the part of the student.
- *Sources of information* available to the student including digital sources have expanded. Students are bombarded with information from a range of sources including lectures, tutorials, small group discussions, practical and clinical classes, textbooks, handouts, apps and the world wide web.
- The introduction of *educational approaches* such as Problem Based Learning and the Flipped Classroom are associated with a greater emphasis on independent learning and have required the student to take more responsibility for their own learning, with greater reliance being placed on the student for effective and efficient information processing.

In this chapter, we outline key features of this role and discuss the opportunities and challenges of information processing and seeking for students. We start by considering how information is processed in the brain and how a student can make this information processing more effective and efficient. We then consider the student's role as an information seeker; what competencies are required, what sources students most often use, and the factors that shape the choices.

While our focus is on the role of the student, it is important to note that it should not be the sole responsibility of the student to develop their information processing strategies. Students are best placed to judge what strategies work best for them, but they should be supported to better understand learning and appropriate strategies for information processing. The curriculum should be designed to facilitate students' information processing and information seeking.

The student as information processor

Information processing is a rapidly advancing field of study, sitting at the crossroads of scientific research and educational practice, with brain researchers, educational psychologists, medical teachers, and students engaged as actors. The simple linear model of input and output to the brain has evolved. We now have a more complex understanding of the brain and how information is processed and recorded in various ways, with the ability to access the information later enhanced. There has also been greater recognition of emotional and motivational factors, and the value students give to their studies has been shown to influence students' information processing (Bruinsma, 2004).

How we process information depends on a number of factors (Mayer, 2010; Pressley et al., 1989).

- The individual's cognitive abilities
- The quantity of information to be remembered
- The student's motivation and how focused they are on processing the information
- The extent to which the student perceives the information as relevant

- How what is being learned is related to what was previously learned
- Repetition and presentation of information in different formats such as text, diagram, and audio

Helping the student to process information

Processing information, one might think, should be easy for a student, given that by this point they have been processing information in an educational context for many years and have demonstrated their ability by gaining entry to medical school. However, this may not be the case, and for the most part, students need guidance in developing strategies which will result in more effective and efficient information processing. Pelley (2014) argued that just as we can improve our body by bodybuilding, so we can also, with appropriate strategies, improve our brain and information processing ability. He noted, "Students who understand how their brain works, always perform better than those who do not".

Humans are processors of information, and the mind is an information-processing system (Mayer, 1996). The learner's thought mechanisms have been equated to that of a computer with information encoded in our memory in a series of stages. Learning is what happens when the brain receives information, records it and stores it for retrieval later from long-term memory (Atkinson and Shiffrin, 1968; Sternberg and Sternberg, 2012) (Figure 6.1).

Information is held, in the first place, in the *sensory memory* for a brief period of time as a copy of what is presented. This process can be seen as acting as a filter by focusing on what is seen as important. The information is then stored for a short time in the *working memory* which has a limited capacity (seven +/− two pieces of information). For example, Ingram (1999) described how bar waiting staff can dramatically increase their memory relating to drinks orders. The executive control system of the working memory oversees active learning and the selection of information from the sensory memory, the processing of the information, and the decision as to whether to transfer the information or not to the long-term memory (Baddeley, 2001).

Unlike working memory, *long-term memory* has unlimited space. Information is available from long-term memory when required. Information is retrieved from the long-term memory to the working memory when it has to be used. This may be to inform decisions in clinical practice, to answer questions at the time of an examination, or to support further learning. A crucial factor in later retrieval is how well the information is organised.

There are several general strategies that can be used by students to improve the processing of information and learning (Marzano, 2009; Mayer, 2010; Cerbin, 2018) (Figure 6.2).

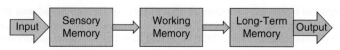

Figure 6.1 The information processing system.

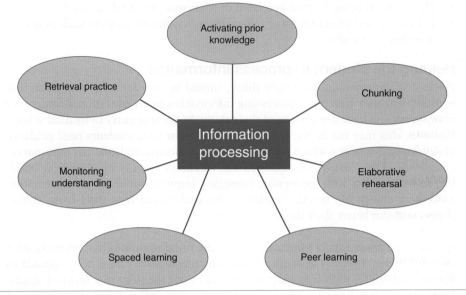

Figure 6.2 Strategies adopted to enhance information processing.

Retrieval practice

Retrieval practice as described by Jones (2019) refers to the act of recalling information from memory. Every time the information is retrieved, the information is cemented in the long-term memory, enabling it to be retrieved more easily in the future. In this way, the act of retrieving information from our memory and bringing it to mind dramatically improves learning (Box 6.1).

Tom Sherrington (2019) argued, "Practicing remembering is at the very core of what effective learning is about. The more often we retrieve knowledge from our vast complex stores of memories in different ways – all those facts, words, ideas, concepts, and experiences – the stronger these memories become and the more fluently we can recall them."

Box 6.1 Demonstration of the value of retrieval practice

From *Karpicke, J.D., Bauernschmidt, A. 2011. Spaced retrieval: Absolute spacing enhances learning regardless of relative spacing. J. Exp. Psychol. Learn. Mem. Cogn. 37 (5), 1250–1257.*

In the study, the student objective was to learn a list of foreign language words and their translation.

The student saw a vocabulary word and had to recall its translation. Once a word was recalled, the student had to practise retrieving it three times, either immediately or at spaced intervals throughout the learning session.

The proportion of words and translations that the student remembered was studied one week later. It was found that the simple addition of spaced retrieval practice took the student's performance from nearly total forgetting to extremely good retention with about 80% correct.

Activating prior knowledge

The student can start a learning session with a brief review of what they have previously learned about the topic. This brings what is in the long-term memory back into the working memory so that new information can be integrated with what has been learned previously. An example is given in Box 6.2.

Chunking

New information can be arranged in small chunks to avoid overloading the working memory. Stopping between the chunks allows time to process the information. An example of chunking is also given in Box 6.2.

Elaborative rehearsal

Elaborative rehearsal involves thinking about the meaning of the information and connecting it with what is already known and stored in the memory. It helps to translate information from the working memory into the long-term memory.

Spaced learning

Spaced learning involves repeated learning of material at intervals, with unrelated material studied in between. This improves memory and retention. It gives the student's mind the opportunity to form connections between ideas and concepts so that knowledge can be built upon and recalled later. Information passes from the working memory to the long-term memory where it can be more easily retrieved later.

Monitoring understanding

It helps if the student continually checks their understanding of what they are learning. The use of end-of-week quizzes can be very helpful in allowing students to test their knowledge. These may be recall questions to test factual knowledge,

---

Box 6.2 An example of information processing strategies as applied to the topic "hyperthyroidism"

The following activities can help one learn and move information about hyperthyroidism from the working to the long-term memory from where it can later be more easily accessed.

The information presented about hyperthyroidism in a lecture or described in a textbook can be broken down into *smaller chunks* of information: the prevalence and importance of the diagnosis; the clinical features; the investigation of thyroid function; treatment with antithyroid drugs; treatment with surgery; treatment with radioactive iodine; and patient-centred care.

The information in a chunk can be used to *activate prior knowledge*, bringing what is in the long-term memory back into the working memory. Examples include the clinical features of hyperthyroidism relating to the physiology of thyroid hormone, the use of antithyroid drugs relating to the biochemistry of thyroid hormone production, and the use of thyroid surgery relating to the anatomy of the thyroid gland.

Thinking about information relating to hyperthyroidism can be *elaborated on and rehearsed* when you see a patient with hyperthyroidism at a clinic or as a virtual patient online. Information processing is also improved if the student *monitors and assesses* their learning by answering questions and problems relating to hyperthyroidism.

but it is better to move beyond recall and encourage students to evaluate their understanding through the application of knowledge. Creating opportunities where students are required to create a question (in class or on a discussion board) is also a good way to encourage them to monitor how well they have understood a topic: it is difficult to formulate a question on a topic in which the student has limited understanding.

Peer learning

Working in groups can lead to more active learning because students can:

- Summarise information and key concepts for other members of the group
- Identify what is confusing
- Question each other

Peer learning has an important role to play when students practise for clinical exams (for example OSCEs). We highlighted the importance of peer learning – collaborative and cooperative – in Chapter 5 and return to this again in later chapters. Box 6.3 presents an innovative collaborative project in which students developed a digital resources to support their own as well as their peers' learning for the Prescribing Safety Assessment (https://prescribingsafetyassessment.ac.uk/).

Box 6.3 Student Case Study: Creating a digital resource to support learning for the Prescribing Safety Assessment

An example of a student-developed digital resource to support learning, by Anna Wijngaard, University of Edinburgh

For my Student Selected Component, a group of peers and I created a digital resource on the Prescribing Safety Assessment (PSA; https://prescribingsafetyassessment.ac.uk). From personal experience in preparing for the assessment, I found multiple resources that were helpful. However, I found myself combining different "official" and unaffiliated or commercial sources, and lacked clarity on the reliability and applicability. When practising drug prescriptions, including dose calculations and monitoring requirements, having up-to-date and accurate information is crucial. I spent a significant amount of time looking for and evaluating resources and processing those into a concise and reliable summary to base my studying. I find that this process can be quite inefficient, but I do actually find myself thinking more about the information I am reading, and the product is very useful for revision purposes.

When we started this project, our aim was to create an accurate, one-stop resource for students on the PSA, to share our learning and abbreviate the process of finding reliable information for other students. By doing more research, we acquired even more detailed knowledge of the assessment and eventually shifted to writing mock questions and workings, which we used in our videos. We purposely chose this format as it would not simply present the information but would also require interaction from the user. We had a rigorous checking process and involved senior staff and doctors, as we wanted to ensure reliability and the practice of evidence-based medicine. The process was challenging and required careful management, but I learned a lot in the end, not only about pharmacology, but also about developing research skills and processing and presenting my findings in a format to aid learning.

Processing information in practice

The strategies designed to improve information processing described above can be applied to learning in a range of contexts, including information presented in the lecture, printed text, and online information. The strategies described may be adapted to suit the different contexts and the student's personal needs. Here we focus on the lecture as one important source of information for the student.

Lectures often present students with particular information processing challenges; the rate of delivery of information via the teacher is often faster than the student can record in their notes. Logan (1991) described nine steps based on information processing theory which, if applied to the lecture, can lead to better information processing. Logan recognised that the optimum learning style will vary from student to student and should be tailored to the student's personal needs. Below we present a modified version of Logan's recommendations. We also consider how recordings of lectures may support these steps towards effective information processing (Nordmann et al., 2022).

Step 1: Prepare

Preparing to process the information in a lecture can begin before the lecture by reviewing notes from the previous lecture: this prepares the mind to start processing new ideas by accessing prior knowledge from the long-term memory. The student familiarising themselves with the content to be covered, in advance, is helped to develop a general framework within which they can organise the information. Such preparation is contingent on the lecture topic and slides being made available with sufficient notice prior to the lecture, and advance notices of teaching slots during clinical placements to allow for such preparation.

Step 2: Active Listening

During the lecture, students should actively engage by listening to the lecturer rather than trying to take extensive notes as writing requires a lot of attention which detracts from listening. Making lecture recordings available to students supports active listening by removing their fear of missing something in their notes. Teachers could remind students of this in class and ensure that students are given advice on how to best use recordings.

Step 3: Review

The ideas learned in a lecture immediately begin to fade from the working memory. As soon as possible after the lecture, students should rewrite their notes while remembering the lecture. This can be useful to organise the ideas into chunks of information. For recorded lectures, this can involve re-watching parts of the lecture that remain unclear. This is part of the elaborative rehearsal described above. By doing this the student has begun to practise the information presented and making it easier to retrieve it later from their long-term memory. With increased use of lecture recordings, greater attention has been given to the amount of time it takes to engage with lecture information. Although it varies by topic and individual student knowledge, students should be allocated double the time of the recording to be able to listen, take notes and review their learning. The time required to review information from lectures should be considered when planning students' weekly timetables.

Step 4: Recite

It can be useful to repeat the information from the lecture in your own words, without referring to notes. This can be done with other students, as part of a study group, and is a powerful learning tool to help information remain in the long-term memory. Lecture recordings can be a very useful resource to help students monitor their understanding as they engage in this recall.

The student as an information seeker

Advances in medical sciences, and changes in disease patterns such as with COVID-19, constantly require new information. Before graduating, students cannot possibly acquire all the information they will need for lifetime practice in medicine. An essential attribute of the graduate is the ability, as an information seeker, to navigate the vast information available to find, access, and evaluate information as it is required or as it becomes available. Patton and Friedman (2017) argued that all students "must learn to be skilled navigators and discriminating users of information".

Information-seeking competencies

As the volume of information available to students has grown exponentially through the internet, increasing attention has been given to the information skills and competencies that graduates should develop. The Colorado Department of Education specified a series of twenty-first-century information literacy skills required of a graduate, as listed in Box 6.4.

Friedman et al. (2016) described three competencies required of the student in relation to their role as an information seeker.

Knowing what you do and do not know

The doctor must be able to recognise when they have incomplete knowledge and have reached the limit of their knowledge competence and require obtaining further information.

> Historically medical education has rewarded students who carry the right answer in their heads. In the informational future, we should instead reward students who understand the flaws and limits in their knowledge, and appropriately manage their uncertainty (Friedman et al., 2016)

The expectation to "carry the right answer in their heads" can create significant pressure for students and may lead to a reluctance by the student to give answers to questions in teaching contexts (whether clinical or in the classroom). One student reported that during their intercalated year, they felt there was a greater openness to

Box 6.4 Student information literacy requirements as recommended by the Colorado Department of Education

From *Colorado Department of Education Graduation Guidelines. Work Group Reports and Recommendations on 21st Century Skills. Colorado Department of Education. Accessed on 17/02/2021 at https://www.cde.state.co.us/postsecondary/21st-century-skills-draft-summary-recommendation.*

- Analyse primary and secondary sources
- Communicate sound reasoning using texts, graphics, and speech
- Curate information from multiple resources
- Evaluate and validate the credibility and relevance of information
- Explore divergent thinking and diverse points of view
- Integrate and apply appropriate technology to access and evaluate new information
- Interpret information critically to detect bias and/or purpose for a target audience
- Synthesize/converge evidence from multiple sources to strengthen arguments

discussion about scientific knowledge, which in turn reduced the pressure to have the right answer. While clearly there is some concreteness in medical knowledge, there is much that is changing, and educators should support students to engage critically with knowledge and to discuss how to learn and practise in the context of uncertainty. This clearly links to the student's role as information processor and the importance of monitoring understanding. We discuss the student's role in assessment in Chapter 8. An interesting account of the importance of this as a skill in clinical practice is given in Box 6.5.

The ability to ask a good question

The process of formulating questions encourages students to reflect on and assess their knowledge, and supports the process of seeking information by identifying areas where they require further information (Taylor, 1962). Students can be supported to do this by embedding opportunities for questions within all teaching and

Box 6.5 Knowledge seeking during uncertainty: critical care consultants in the COVID-19 pandemic

From *Sawyer, R., Harden, J., Baruah, R. 2022 Intensive care clinicians' information acquisition during the first wave of the Covid 19 pandemic. J. Intensive Care Soc. Epub ahead of print. https://doi.org/10.1177/17511437221105777.*

Critical care consultants faced significant challenges acquiring and evaluating information to guide clinical decision making during the first wave of the COVID-19 pandemic. A qualitative study with critical care consultants revealed that clinicians were profoundly affected by the ways in which the pandemic changed, in a very short space of time, how they could access information to guide clinical decision-making. Peer-reviewed journals were perceived as less reliable sources given the speed at which the situation was changing. Two strategies were adopted to address the urgent need for, yet paucity of reliable information on the virus – an organised approach to data collection across the wider critical care community and the establishment of a local community of collaborative decision-making. This flexible and pragmatic approach to information acquisition seemed to provide reassurance to participants by giving some local standardisation to clinical decision-making until trials of COVID-19 therapies were able to report their findings.

learning contexts. This may be as simple as giving time in class for students to formulate a question or may be at the heart of the teaching approach, for example, through inquiry-based teaching or problem-based learning.

Evaluating and weighing the evidence

The ability to identify and evaluate research evidence to improve clinical practice and patient care is central to becoming a good doctor. This is a key principle in evidence-based medicine (EBM), which is now commonly addressed in the medical curriculum (Albarqouni et al., 2018). There are challenges for students in learning and practising EBM including sub-optimal role models, an unwillingness to show uncertainty, time constraints and space in the curriculum to allow for critical discussion, and dislocation of EBM from clinical contexts (Maggio et al., 2016). However, Nicholson et al. (2020) found that despite challenges, students are able to identify, evaluate, and effectively use sources to answer clinical questions.

What information sources are used and for what purpose?

Specific sources used by students are likely to change, but current research indicates that students consult a range of resources: expert point-of-care sources such as *Epocrates* and *UpToDate*; more generalised sources such as *Google* and *Wikipedia*; databases such as PubMed; and textbooks (Twiss-Brooks et al., 2017; Ryan et al., 2020). It may be of some concern that sites that are not considered trustworthy sources of information (such as Wikipedia) are used. However, there is evidence that even when students begin a search using such sources, they are aware of their lack of trustworthiness and tend to use them as a gateway to more reliable sources (Nicholson et al., 2020). Information from such sources is used for immediate learning, for example, to follow up on patient care and clinical issues including diagnosis and drug dosing information.

Question banks

Question banks (such as Passmedicine, Pastest, and Quesmed) are also commonly used to practise many of the learning strategies discussed earlier: indeed, many draw on an understanding of information processing in the development of their learning tools. For example, flashcards and knowledge summaries allow students to practise, assess, and re-assess their knowledge while identifying areas of weakness. It is worth noting that many such question banks require payment, thereby creating an inequity in access to learning resources. To address this, medical schools can consider offering financial support to students who may otherwise not be able to afford access to a question bank. A more inclusive approach would involve the school subscribing to question banks at an institutional level, giving automatic access to all their students. In Box 6.6, we present a student case study describing one such question bank and the links to accessing learning via social media platforms.

Free Open Access Medicine and social media

Free Open Access Medical education (FOAM) can facilitate students' access to the most up-to-date research findings and discussion of clinical practice, for example

Box 6.6 Student case study: social media and question banks

An example of the use of social media and a question bank by Priyesh Agravat, University College London

Having run the social media accounts (primarily Instagram and Facebook) of the medical question bank Quesmed for the past 18 months, one of the main things I have learnt is the increasing role of social media in medical education. While university resources should theoretically cover the majority of the curricula in a digestible and easy-to-access variety of formats, this is not always the case, and not everybody learns the same way. For many, the use of an extensive question bank with flashcards that use spaced repetition (something most universities cannot offer) as a means to learn is a much more effective way of learning than the more "traditional method" of listening to a consultant go through a 100+ slide presentation with little interaction.

Quesmed uses novel methods of learning such as daily questions and flashcards on their social media accounts, which combined can reach well over 10,000 accounts every day. This captures the true value of opportunistic learning via social media. Even if students are online and expecting to browse memes or see what their friends are up to, they could instead pick up a fact or two that might just gain them those extra marks in their finals.

Quesmed was one of the first to provide live, interactive, free-to-attend online lectures at the start of the pandemic when most medical schools effectively "closed" and ended in-person placements and teaching. These were widely received and viewed internationally, sometimes attended by over 1000 students. They now have an offline mobile app which has a searchable textbook covering all core conditions that a medical student would need to know, as well as the main question bank function, a resource most universities do not provide, that makes learning on the go that bit more convenient.

Even before the COVID-19 pandemic, it would be unheard of for a student to only use university resources to pass exams, but there is an increasing reliance on non-university resources now more than ever as medical schools across the world adjust how they deliver education. The role of social media will continue to grow in this space and become a more integral part of the medical school experience.

through open-access journals, and time-limited free access to subscription journals. Much of the conversation arising from FOAM happens via social media and as such there are some risks – the information may not yet have undergone peer review and the discussion and comments arising from it may cause confusion for students as multiple experts in the field offer differing opinions. Equally, the information accessed via FOAM may differ from that being taught in class. One student told us that they learn the Cockcroft Gault/eGFR equations for exams as still accounting for race, whereas FOAM resources they had accessed disputed this (for example, http://www.nephjc.com/news/raceandegfr). This can be exciting and enlightening if students are supported in engaging with and using such sources in their learning. Indeed, it may be useful to bring such conversations directly into the classroom to connect to real-world debates in science and clinical practice and to help students develop skills in navigating social media as a learning resource.

Factors in selection and use of information resources

The most commonly cited factors that influence the resources student use are the speed and convenience of access. In clinical settings, students often have limited time to find information, and in non-clinical contexts, workload pressures mean that students favour time-efficient approaches to studying. This leads to a preference for resources that are easy to access, for example, those that do not require repeated logins and are organised logically, making them easy to use. Connected to this, students prefer resources that are accessible and easy to view on portable electronic devices such as smartphones and tablets. Studies have suggested near-universal ownership of such devices by medical students, providing them with flexible and immediate access to online resources (Chase et al., 2018).

Social factors have also been reported as influencing students' information-seeking. Twiss-Brooks et al. (2017) describe this as "putting on the white coat", referring to what was considered appropriate contexts for information seeking. Students have expressed concern about using their smartphones to search for information during clinical encounters in case patients or clinicians view this negatively. This may relate to concerns about phone use visibly demonstrating a knowledge gap or potential confusion over why the phone was being used (for example, for personal communication rather than seeking essential information). However, Chase et al. (2018) did not report such concerns, perhaps signalling a shift as smartphones become increasingly embedded and accepted in all aspects of everyday and professional life.

Conclusion

Information is processed in the brain in working memory and long-term memory. Information processing efficiency can be improved by adopting strategies such as retrieval practice, activating prior knowledge, chunking, elaborative rehearsal, spaced learning, monitoring understanding and peer learning.

A range of information processing strategies can be adopted in different contexts, for example, in relation to the lecture. There is no one-size-fits-all strategy: the optimum information processing strategy can be tailored to the needs of the individual student and the specific context in which they are learning.

Increasingly there are expectations that students should not only be an information processor but also an information seeker. In this role, they need to identify what they need to know, identify possible sources of information; and evaluate the information they retrieve.

References

Albarqouni, L., Hoffmann, T., Glasziou, P., 2018. Evidence-based practice educational intervention studies: A systematic review of what is taught and how it is measured. BMC Med. Educ. 18, 177.

Atkinson, R.C., Shiffrin, R.M., 1968. Human memory: A proposed system and its control processes. Psychol. Learn. Motiv. 2, 89–195.

Baddeley, A.D., 2001. Is working memory still working? Am. Psychol. 56 (11), 851–864.

Bruinsma, M., 2004. Motivation, cognitive processing and achievement in higher education. Learn. Instruct. 14 (6), 549–568.

Cerbin, W., 2018. Improving student learning from lectures. Scholarsh Teach. Learn. Psychol. 4 (3), 151–163.

Chase, T.J.G., Julius, A., Chandan, J.S., Powell, E., Hall, C.S., Phillips, B.L., Burnett, R., Gill, D., Fernando, B., 2018. Mobile learning in medicine: An evaluation of attitudes and behaviours of medical students. BMC Med. Educ. 18 (1), 152.

Colorado Department of Education Graduation Guidelines. Work Group Reports and Recommendations on 21st Century Skills. Colorado Department of Education. Accessed on 17/02/2021 at https://www.cde.state.co.us/postsecondary/21st-century-skills-draft-summary-recommendation.

Friedman, C.P., Donaldson, K.M., Vantsevich, A.V., 2016. Educating medical students in the era of ubiquitous information. Med. Teach. 38 (5), 504–509.

Gibney, E., 2014. How to tame the flood of literature. Nature. 513, 129–130.

Harden, R.M., Lilley, P.M., 2018. The Eight Roles of the Medical Teacher. Elsevier, London, UK.

Ingram, J., 1999. The Barmaid's Brain and Other Strange Tales from Science. Ourum Press, London, UK.

Jones, K., 2019. Retrieval Practice. John Catt Educational Ltd, Suffolk, UK.

Karpicke, J.D., Bauernschmidt, A., 2011. Spaced retrieval: Absolute spacing enhances learning regardless of relative spacing. J. Exp. Psychol. Learn. Mem. Cogn. 37 (5), 1250–1257.

Logan, F.A., 1991. Learning from lectures. In: College Learning: Ways and Whys. Kendall Hunt Publishing, Dubuque, Iowa, USA.

Maggio, L.A., ten Cate, O., Chen, H.C., Irby, D.M., O'Brien, B.C., 2016. Challenges to learning evidence-based medicine and educational approaches to meet these challenges: A qualitative study of selected EBM curricula in U.S. and Canadian medical schools. Acad. Med. 91, 101–106.

Marzano, R., 2009. The art and science of teaching/helping students process information. Educ. Lead. 67, 86–87.

Mayer, R., 1996. Learners as information processors: Legacies and limitations of educational psychology's second metaphor. Educ. Psychol. 31 (3), 151–161.

Mayer, R.E., 2010. Applying the science of learning to medical education. Med. Educ. 44 (6), 543–549.

Nicholson, J., Kalet, A., van der Vleuten, C., de Bruin, A., 2020. Understanding medical student evidence-based medicine information seeking in an authentic clinical simulation. J. Med. Libr. Assoc. 108 (2), 219–228.

Nordmann, E., Kuepper-Tetzel, C.E., Robson, L., Phillipson, S., Lipan, G.I., McGeorge, P., 2022. Lecture capture: Practical recommendations for students and lecturers. Scholarsh. Teach. Learn. Psychol. 8(3),174–193. https://doi.org/10.1037/stl0000190.

Patton, C., Friedman, C.P., 2017. Medical education in an era of ubiquitous information. In: Dent, J.A., Harden, R.M., Hunt, D. (Eds.), A Practical Guide for Medical Teachers (5th ed). Elsevier, London, UK.

Pelley, J., 2014. Body building for the brain. TEDtalk. Accessed on 10/2/22 at https://www.youtube.com/watch?v=3Roz6BVdKcQ.

Pressley, M., Borkwski, J.G., Schneider, W., 1989. Chapter 2: Good information processing: what it is and how education can promote it. Int. J. Educ. Res. 13 (8), 857–867.

Ryan, L., Sheehan, K., Marion, M.I., Harbison, J., 2020. Online resources used by medical students, a literature review. MedEdPublish. 9, 136. https://doi.org/10.15694/mep.2020.000136.1.

Sawyer, R., Harden, J., Baruah, R., 2022. Intensive care clinicians' information acquisition during the first wave of the Covid 19 pandemic. J. Intensive Care Soc. Epub ahead of print. https://doi.org/10.1177/17511437221105777.

Sherrington, T., 2019. Foreword. In: Jones, K. (Ed.), Retrieval Practice. John Catt Education Ltd, Suffolk, UK, pp. 13.

Sternberg, R.J., Sternberg, K., 2012. Cognitive Psychology. Wadsworth, Cengage Learning, Belmont, CA, USA, pp. 212–213, 193–205.

Taylor, R.S., 1962. The process of asking questions. Amer. Doc. 13, 391–396.

Twiss-Brooks, A.B., Andrade Jr, R., Bass, M.B., Kern, B., Peterson, J., Werner, D.A., 2017. A day in the life of third-year medical students: Using an ethnographic method to understand information seeking and use. J. Med. Libr. Assoc. 105 (1), 12–19.

The student as a curriculum collaborator   7

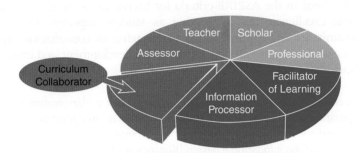

The student's role

Students as partners? This might raise some eyebrows! After all, aren't teachers there to teach and students there to learn? Well I have found that this could not be further from the truth. I experienced the benefits of student-staff collaboration when I participated in a two-week project for year one MBBS curriculum redesign at the Imperial College School of Medicine (ICSM) in 2019. We produced output that led to significant changes in the curriculum in the short space of two weeks (SJ Kapadia, 2021, a student at Imperial Medical School in the UK).

The concept of curriculum negotiation was developed by Gareth Boomer in the 1980s (Bron et al., 2016). Boomer et al. (1992, p. 10) argued that students have a role in decisions about the curriculum, with the curriculum seen as a process instead of a predetermined externally established product. There should be a shared, detailed understanding between teachers and students of what is going on, what needs to be done, and how it will be done. Boomer described the negotiations of the curriculum as

The deliberate planning to invite students to contribute to and to modify the educational programme so that they will have a real investment, both in the learning journey and in the outcome.

Student engagement with the curriculum, contributing to design, management, and evaluation, is the cornerstone of the concept of students as partners in the education programme. Cook-Sather et al. (2014, pp. 6–7) defined student partnership in curriculum development as

> *A collaborative reciprocal process through which all participants have the opportunity to contribute equally, although not necessarily in the same ways, to curricular or pedagogical conceptualisation, decision making, implementation, investigations, or analyses.*

The contribution students can make to the curriculum, in their role as a curriculum evaluator and as a member of a curriculum committee, is well established. These are described in the ASPIRE criteria for Excellence in Student Engagement (www.aspire-to-excellence.org). By serving as student representatives on programme committees, and by instigating or engaging in consultations regarding governance issues, students can play a part in the development and enactment of school policies.

> *Through co-creation, teachers and learners get a better understanding of each other's perspectives on education. This can facilitate a more positive, inclusive and democratic learning environment, increased internal motivation, and higher quality of the educational design* (Könings et al., 2021).

Many teachers, however, may find the idea of students as curriculum co-creators more difficult to accept because it challenges ingrained beliefs that the teacher is there to teach (including developing the curriculum) and that the student is there to learn (Kapadia, 2021). To adapt Jean Brodie, "for those who believe that sort of thing, that is the sort of thing they will believe".

In whatever way students are involved as a curriculum collaborator, there is a potential change in the student/teacher power dynamics. As noted by Bryson (2014), there is

> *A change in the position of the student and the teacher: a more democratic relationship where the student's view is drawn on and valued, and the teacher's role changes to facilitator and becoming a co-learner (p. 236).*

However, such a change does not happen automatically when students are involved as curriculum collaborators, and we need to consider carefully what is intended by partnerships, how this is enacted in practice and how best we can ensure that students' involvement is meaningful.

In this chapter, we consider and explore the student's role as a curriculum collaborator through their involvement (Figure 7.1) in:

- Evaluating the curriculum
- Serving as a member of a curriculum committee
- Co-creating the curriculum

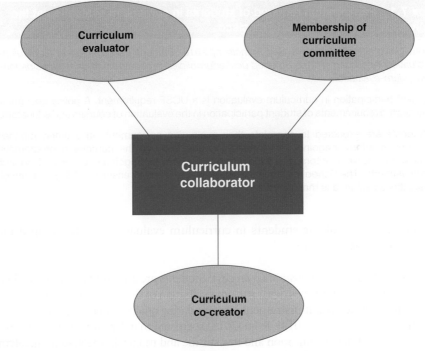

Figure 7.1 Three aspects of the student as curriculum collaborator.

The student as a curriculum evaluator

In response to pressures from the different stakeholders, including the public, employing organisations, accrediting bodies and students as key actors in the process, evaluation of the curriculum is high on today's agenda in medical education (Tang et al., 2012).

The evaluation of the curriculum has a number of functions and associated benefits:

- Self-assessment by the school with a view to, where necessary, improve the functioning of the curriculum
- Validation of the curriculum for an external accrediting body
- Recognition of the importance of teaching through making explicit teaching and curriculum priorities
- Support and encouragement for appropriate changes in the curriculum and broader educational strategies

That students have a role to play in the evaluation of the curriculum is widely accepted, although their precise role may be disputed. For some, this role may be an expectation, whereas in other medical schools it may be a more formal requirement, as described in Box 7.1 for the University of California San Francisco.

Box 7.1 Participation required of students in curriculum evaluation at the University of California, San Francisco

From *University of California San Francisco, 2018. Student Participation in Curriculum Evaluation. Accessed at https://meded.ucsf.edu/policies-procedures/student-participation-curriculum-evaluation*

Student participation in curriculum evaluation is a UCSF requirement. A policy document outlines the requirements of student participation in the evaluation of courses and educators.

"Students are expected to complete their evaluation assignments in a timely manner in order to inform ongoing decision-making and improve the curriculum programme educators, course directors, and educational leadership for ongoing decision making and improvements. The School of Medicine makes every effort to ensure that the quantity of evaluations assigned is manageable for students".

The benefits of involving students in curriculum evaluation can be grouped into two categories (Ryan, 2015):

- *Benefits to the quality assurance process:* Students are an essential part of quality assurance of programmes, with student evaluation of the academic programme serving as a significant instrument for stimulating quality enhancement in a university (Stukalina, 2014). Ryan (2015) suggested that "given that students are the centre of higher education and invest time and money in the system, involving them is important and can improve the QA process". From an accountability perspective, student evaluation helps to hold teachers, programme teams and schools accountable for their performance in enhancing students' education.
- *Benefits to the student:* Serving as a curriculum evaluator results in the development of professional skills including giving constructive feedback. It can also contribute towards the student's sense of ownership of the education programme.

Evidence of teaching effectiveness

Berk (2013) described twelve sources of evidence of teaching effectiveness and advocated triangulating three or more different sources of evidence, so that the strengths of one source can compensate for the weaknesses of another, providing a more accurate, reliable and comprehensive picture of teaching effectiveness. Students are responsible for providing evidence in a number of the approaches (Box 7.2).

Student ratings

In practice, student ratings of courses and teachers have dominated as the primary, and sometimes the only, measure of teaching effectiveness in medical schools. A questionnaire that asks students to rate the different aspects of the teaching and learning programmes on a standard 4- or 5-point scale, perhaps with additional free-text responses, is widely seen as a proxy for a direct measure of the value of the student's learning experience. Despite, or perhaps because of, their prevalence, there is considerable discussion around the use of such questionnaires in terms of validity and reliability, and on the impact of the results on the curriculum. There have been more than 2000 references published on the topic of the educational effectiveness of rating scales (Berk, 2013), with the first article published 90 years ago (Freyd, 1923).

> **Box 7.2** 12 sources of evidence of teaching effectiveness (Berk, 2013)
>
> From *Berk, R.A., 2013. Top five flashpoints in the assessment of teaching effectiveness. Med. Teach. 35 (1), 15–26.*
>
> - Student ratings
> - Peer observations
> - Peer review of course material
> - External expert ratings
> - Self ratings
> - Videos
> - Student interviews
> - Teaching scholarship
> - Administrator ratings
> - Teaching portfolios
> - Alumni ratings
> - Employer ratings

There are concerns about low student response rates and the resulting impact on the reliability and validity of the data. Students have other priorities and may be reluctant to devote the necessary time and thought to the evaluation process. Some argue that there are behaviours and skills defining teaching effectiveness which students might not be able to rate based on their experiences: for example, it may not be possible to evaluate a teacher's knowledge and expertise based on a single or even several teaching sessions. Ratings may also be susceptible to a halo effect where a high rating on one aspect might influence the student to rate other unrelated items highly. For example, enthusiastic teachers tend to receive more favourable ratings on all criteria, even when the content is flawed (Schiekirka et al., 2015). A randomised controlled trial with medical students found that the students given chocolate cookies evaluated teachers significantly better than those who did not receive the cookies (Hessler et al., 2018). The chocolate itself may have improved the mood of students, or perhaps the offering of the cookies made the students feel valued. Such research highlights that multiple factors can influence students' evaluations of teaching.

Concerns have also been raised regarding bias and prejudice in students' evaluations arising from the race, gender, age and nationality of the student and the teacher (Heffernan, 2022). A study of 43,000 course evaluations by Tucker et al., (2014) found that across every discipline and course, evaluations submitted by women were overall two per cent more favourable. Fan et al. (2019), in a study of 22,000 evaluations, found that male students express a significant bias in favour of male teachers. Some have investigated gender bias via the use of avatars in online learning and found that male avatars (regardless of the teacher behind the avatar's gender) are more highly rated than female avatars (MacNell, Driscoll, and Hunt, 2015). The results of the research are also concerning in relation to ethnicity, language, and perceptions of sexuality or disability, with evidence of prejudice in student evaluations (Heffernan, 2022). For example, people from minority ethnic backgrounds, and/or who do not speak English as their first language, are evaluated less positively (Fan et al., 2019).

Improving student evaluation questionnaires

Despite the concerns noted above, student ratings remain cost-effective, time efficient, and are considered to be adequate in terms of reliability for a given teacher and course (Little et al., 2009; Berk, 2013). Beyond the issues of validity and reliability, there is value in retaining student ratings of teaching (and their educational experience) as one means to provide all students with the opportunity to express their opinions on their educational experiences.

There are a number of factors to consider when seeking to improve student evaluation questionnaires that may help to address some of the issues raised above:

- *Explain the quality assurance process:* To encourage students to respond to course or programme evaluations, and staff to participate in preparing and reviewing evaluations, it can be useful to explain the process for reviewing the questionnaires, and how this fits within wider quality assurance processes.
- *Clarity of purpose:* It is important to consider the purpose of the evaluation, for example, whether it is intended to provide data on the organisation and structure of teaching, the performance of the teacher, or both. This will help guide the questions being asked to ensure that the data gathered will be fit for the purpose. Students can help to design and pilot the questions.
- *Keep the dialogue open:* Student evaluations can become part of an ongoing dialogue between students and the programme team. It is important to report back to students on what has been or will be done, or why actions cannot be taken, following student feedback. There may at times be reasons why concerns are not immediately addressed, and often student evaluations can offer completely contrasting positions – the tutorials were the best/worst part of the course – that make it difficult to determine actions to address comments. Nevertheless, it is essential to communicate what actions have been taken or provide explanations for why something suggested or requested by students has not been done. Some schools have adopted "You Said, We Did" or "You Said, We Listened" campaigns to promote changes, developments, and responses to student feedback.
- *Administration of questionnaire:* Administration of rating scales has moved from a printed to an online format. While there may be an initial drop in response rates compared to the gathering of paper copies in person at the end of a session, the benefits of online administration include ease of administration, low cost, and rapid turnaround for processing the results. Online questionnaires also give students more time to consider responses to open-ended items and so may yield more frequent and thoughtful comments. There is no universal agreement as to the best time to administer a questionnaire to maximise response rates, whether immediately at the end of the course or following the course examination.
- *Anonymity:* One issue is whether the student respondent should be required to identify themselves. The reasons for anonymity are obvious, including a concern that a student who rates the teaching badly may be penalised. Under the cloak of anonymity, however, student responses may be unnecessarily harsh or comments may be inappropriate, focusing on personal characteristics—for example, a teacher's appearance, rather than the quality of teaching. For example, one study analysed comments in student evaluations given on the anonymous *Rate My Professor* (RMP) website: 10.6% of comments referred

to the female teacher's appearance, whereas there were no comments on the appearance of the male teacher. It is interesting that in formal university evaluations for the course, no comments were made about appearance of either the female or male teacher (Mitchell and Martin, 2018). This highlights the importance of the context of evaluations and the perception of anonymity, which was likely to be considered greater on RMP. Despite this concern, a study comparing open and anonymous course ratings found there was no significant difference in overall assigned ratings (Alfonso et al., 2005). While it is not clear what impact anonymity has on students' comments, we suggest that maintaining anonymity is important and that training students to provide good feedback can mitigate some of the potentially negative consequences.

- *Train students to give feedback:* Just as teachers are given training in how to provide effective feedback to students, students should be advised on how to give feedback to teachers, what they should be looking for when rating their experience, and how they can best provide narrative feedback that will be helpful and contribute to improvements in the course or programme. This would help to address some of the issues raised above and improve students' sense of responsibility in the process. It would also serve as useful training for students in giving peer feedback, and in their later role providing supervisory feedback. Once training is established, it would also be useful to involve senior students as peer trainers.
- *Reduce the potential for bias:* There are opportunities to mitigate bias when designing an evaluation questionnaire and when training students to give teacher feedback. Research has shown that even minor changes to wording and advice given to students can reduce the impact of gender bias on student ratings (Peterson et al., 2019).

Student curriculum review teams

As an alternative to (or alongside) training all students and gathering individual feedback, a student curriculum review team (SCRT) may be used. An SCRT was established at Johns Hopkins University School of Medicine in 2012 to lead the curriculum improvement process (Kumar et al., 2020). The Johns Hopkins faculty found that the SCRT added value beyond the basic course evaluation. The success of the approach was attributed to the dynamic interactions in describing a course's shortcomings and suggested avenues for improvement through the exchange of views at large class "Town Hall meetings," which focused on the strengths of the course and on areas for improvement. Individuals also had a separate opportunity to express their opinions.

Membership of the curriculum committee

While all students can be engaged in evaluating the curriculum as described above, a small number of students may have a particular input by serving as members of the curriculum committee. In the majority of medical schools, a curriculum committee is responsible for monitoring and evaluating the standards of the education programme. In some contexts, students have a formal role in a medical school curriculum committee (Steyer et al., 2003). Schools vary in student committee membership, and students may be expected to engage with the work of the curriculum committee in different ways.

Student representation

Students serving on committees represent the student body as a whole. However, there is a tension between participative and representative democracy; the distance that may exist between the representation and the student body as a whole (Bryson, 2014, p. 239). To meet the needs of the student engagement model, all students should feel that their views are reflected by their representative on the curriculum committee. The school should have transparent and fair processes for appointing student representatives, part of whose role may be to sit on the curriculum committee. One challenge with student membership is the transient nature of the membership, with students appointed usually for only one or two years. Bryson (2014, p. 240), however, saw this as an advantage with "the regular injection of fresh ideas".

Students' role on the curriculum committee

The requirements of a student committee member may include:

- The ability of the student to commit to regular attendance at meetings
- A commitment to review all papers provided with the agenda prior to the meeting
- A commitment to seek the views of the body of students they are representing and to keep them appraised about the curriculum issues raised and the work of the curriculum committee

Students' representation may be a token one with the students having little or no say in the work of the committee, or students may take a lead in certain aspects of or in the working of the committee as a whole. In practice the students' roles and level of involvement may vary from school to school:

- The students contribute at a meeting of the curriculum committee only when invited to do so
- Students are invited to all meetings, and speak to items on the agenda, but do not bring forward motions before the committee for consideration
- Students propose items for inclusion on the committee's agenda and introduce the items at the committee meeting
- Students vote on curriculum issues raised
- Students lead the curriculum committee

Students have a legitimate interest and will be able to offer a useful opinion on matters relating to the curriculum discussed at committee meetings such as:

- Proposals for curriculum change, such as the inclusion of new topics and alterations in educational strategies
- A report from the assessment committee on overall class performance with areas identified where there is a concern with the assessment process or areas where students have performed poorly
- Elective options available for students
- The school's quality assurance and accreditation process
- Equality, diversity, and inclusion in the curriculum
- The use of technology, including simulation and online learning

The student input in the discussion of these issues can help to ensure that the curriculum meets the expanding demand for flexibility and responsiveness to the needs of an increasingly diverse student body.

Ensuring meaningful involvement of student representatives

When compared to the other roles, the role of students on curriculum committees is perhaps the furthest from the traditional student role. While it may be common for student representatives to sit on committees, it may be considered more challenging to involve students in decision-making. There is a need for consideration of the format and working of the committee to ensure that it is inclusive and facilitates the meaningful participation of students. How students' time and effort are recognised and rewarded should be considered (Crawford, 2012). Students are often not paid for their contribution as representatives on curriculum committees meaning that involvement in such a role, and indeed a representation of the study body, is skewed towards those who can afford the time to do unpaid work. Similar issues have been raised in relation to the involvement of patients and the public (PPI) in medical research committees and in medical education. In both student involvement and PPI contexts, existing hierarchies can inhibit the participation of those who have not traditionally played a significant role.

It is essential, therefore, to consider the format of meetings and the ways in which student contributions are sought, the roles that staff and students have within the committee, and the involvement of students in work that happens between meetings. There may at times be some tension within the curriculum committee resulting from the different perspectives of the students and faculty members. Such differences may result in a productive discussion; however, it is important to avoid falling back on traditional hierarchies, with student views given less weight than those of staff.

Addressing such hierarchies can be challenging for teachers and students. It can be difficult for staff to reflect on ways of working that are taken for granted and established practices of the curriculum committee. While students can be encouraged to raise concerns and make suggestions about their involvement, it may be daunting for them to suggest revisions to the governance structures and their roles within them. It is therefore incumbent on the faculty team to reflect on the form and level of involvement of students in the curriculum committee, whether this best meets the aims and values of the school, and whether and in what way change is needed. This may lead to a reconfiguration of student representatives' involvement beyond the committee structure. For example, Harvard Medical School initiated the Ed Reps programme to gather "real-time" feedback from students

> *With the aim of fostering a culture that promoted a greater sense of partnership between faculty and students for continuous and real-time curricular improvement (Scott et al., 2019)*

Two student case studies (Box 7.3 and 7.4) reflect on the challenges and benefits of involvement in student representative roles.

THE STUDENT AS A CURRICULUM COLLABORATOR

Box 7.3 Promoting change as a student representative

An example of the experience and challenges of being a student representative by Vassili Crispi, Hull York Medical School

Promoting change has probably been one of the toughest challenges in my roles as a student representative and Chair of the Student Staff Committee at Hull York Medical School and as Deputy Chair for Education for Medical Students Committee at the British Medical Association. Whilst in the former I have worked alongside colleagues and staff members to revise our local syllabus; the latter provided me with an appreciation of the vast, complex, and sometimes frustrating relationships between stakeholders which can bring about innovation and change.

Change is often difficult to bring about, especially in systems such as medical education, which have rarely undergone significant alterations. In the United Kingdom, medical education and its mode of delivery have been relatively stagnant for the past 50 years. As a student representative, my greatest accomplishment was leading the drafting and approval of the Joint Policy on Student Representation, providing a stronger, collaborative delivery framework for student representation within my medical school.

Within these roles, my greatest obstacle was finding the confidence to speak truth to power, especially when no one else did. Students who take up positions of representation are often entering an unknown environment where a different, technical language is spoken; this can exclude them from discussions and make them stand out for their inexperience. However, I believe this is a fault of the system, which fails to introduce students to financial and managerial fields earlier on during their school education.

I believe higher education and the NHS fail to recognise the invaluable role that healthcare students can play in driving change. Whilst the focus is placed on studying and service provision, students and trainees are often discouraged from stepping into positions of leadership early on in their careers. I am confident that students and trainees alongside institutions are becoming more aware of the key role of leadership in bringing about change.

The student as a curriculum co-creator

A third role for the student as a curriculum collaborator is the role of the student as a curriculum co-creator. Bovill et al. (2016, p. 196) described co-creation as occurring "when staff and students work collaboratively with one another to create components of curricula and/or pedagogical approaches."

Englander and colleagues (2020) have argued that the educational model should change in line with the healthcare model. In medicine, there has been increasing emphasis on the patient-centred healthcare delivery model, with patients as partners in their healthcare. The authors posit that education, like healthcare services, should follow a service-dominant logic

Like the relationship between patient and providers, the relationship between learner and teacher requires the integrated expertise of each method in the context of their system, community, and society to optimise outcome.

The authors argue that

Health professions learners cannot be educated in a traditional paternalistic model of education and then expected to practice in a manner that prioritises co-productive partnership with colleagues, patients, and families.

Box 7.4   Being Convenor of the Medical Students' Council

An example of the experience of involvement in the Medical Students' Council by Aya Riad, Edinburgh Medical School

I acted as the Convenor of the Medical Students' Council. This involved chairing monthly meetings of our 30-person committee of student representatives, being the first point of contact for students and staff when things go wrong and being in a lot of meetings where I was the youngest and least experienced person.

The best piece of advice I received, that I kept going back to, was that while it can be intimidating to be "just" a student in big meetings, and it is, it's also your superpower – it means they can't ignore you, you are the leading expert on being a student in that room. However, I learnt it does you well to acknowledge that staff have been doing this for a long time; seek to understand the reasoning behind the status quo before demanding change – listen and learn as well as advocate.

The student-facing aspect of the role is perhaps the most rewarding, but it is often difficult to explain to peers the "Feedback – Change Gap" – just because I express a view doesn't mean it will happen; representatives ultimately don't make the decisions. Looking back, I think the most important thing is to speak to as many people as possible and often. To be the only student inputting on decisions means you have to represent every student, and the reality is that most people don't engage with student representation, so you have to actively seek them out.

Taking on this role was the steepest learning curve I experienced, while it was by no means easy it greatly increased my negotiation and leadership skills and confidence. You are capable of enacting change as a student representative. It often won't be dramatic or instantaneous but rather slow and steady – but it will seep through, and that's all that matters.

Students can usefully work with teachers as co-creators of a curriculum, or module within a curriculum. Students and faculty may have different expertise, and for co-creation to be effective and yield maximum benefits, both must appreciate the different perspectives they bring.

Co-creation of the curriculum and the partnership between staff and students, Bovill (2013, p. 464) suggests

> *Is not about giving students complete control, nor is it about staff maintaining complete control…the relative levels of control over decision making and appropriate levels of partnership are likely to depend upon the context, the level of study, the relative experience levels of the students and the staff, the attitudes of students and staff, what is being discussed, and the level of influence of professional bodies over the curriculum.*

Key features of co-creation (Bovill, 2020, p. 31) include an emphasis on:

- Shared goals
- Shared decision-making
- Negotiation
- Valuing student perspectives
- Shared respect
- Shared responsibility
- Reciprocity

The focus for the curriculum co-creation

- *Course/module co-creation:* The focus for the collaboration may range from an element within a course to a complete course, including the learning outcomes, teaching, learning methods, and assessment. It may be the case that such partnerships are responses to gaps identified by staff or students, or in response to wider changes in curricular content. In Box 7.5, we present a student case study describing a staff-student collaboration to create a climate change and sustainability course. The involvement of students in course co-creation can also be embedded in the course organisation. In Box 7.6, we present a student's reflections on the role of "student module co-directors".
- *Curriculum themes/strands:* The collaboration may also relate to a theme running through the education programme, for example, the development of interprofessional education courses (Behrend et al., 2019). Harden and Fawkner (2019) describe the staff-student partnership to develop teaching on physical activity for health: students led the development of resources for flipped classroom sessions including video interviews and cases for discussion.

Box 7.5 Co-creating an "Interdisciplinary Introduction to Climate Change & Sustainability" course

An example of student involvement in co-creating a course by Vidya Nanthakumar, University of Glasgow

Despite being declared the greatest threat to humankind by the World Health Organisation, few medical schools sufficiently teach about the health consequences of the climate crisis. Furthermore, although the climate crisis is an interdisciplinary issue, requiring collaboration across fields to create solutions, in streamlining students by subject, the UK education system results in many STEM students lacking awareness of issues such as the climate crisis.

Noting this, a friend and I, through the University of Glasgow Green New Deal movement, set up the first staff-student collaboratively created, accredited "Interdisciplinary Introduction to Climate Change & Sustainability" evening course at the University of Glasgow. This introduces the causes, consequences, and potential solutions for the climate crisis through an interdisciplinary lens. We hoped the course would be accessible to all as it was in the evenings, only 10 credits, and available to be audited (taken without credits for degrees with a maximum mandatory credit requirement, e.g., medicine). In the first run of the course in January 2021, it proved successful, with 49 students from all years and most subjects represented!

There were, however, challenges in starting this. Until we received "official" support from University lecturers, we sent countless emails to anyone we thought could help – a tiring and demotivating process. Furthermore, despite setting up a course being simple in theory, the lack of transparency in navigating this process and knowing who to contact, meant a lot of time and energy was spent at this stage. I also became aware of the lack of spaces existing to collaborate with staff on addressing curricular issues, specifically socio-political ones. This issue is amplified in medical schools where medicine is often (wrongly) framed as separate from the socio-political context it is situated within. Initiatives like the "Planetary Health Report Card" are therefore vital in creating collaborative spaces and staff-student networks invested in specific issues.

These experiences highlighted the developments that can be made when staff and students work together to push for change, with students bringing original, "out of the box" ideas and staff providing the inside bureaucratic knowledge to make these ideas a credible reality. I hope the networks of staff and students interested in creating curricular change on the climate crisis created through this project will remain in place for future generations of medical students and that this can provide a foundation for future collaboration.

Box 7.6 Experience as a student module co-director

An example of student co-creation in curriculum management by Hannes Kruger and colleagues, medical students at Charité – Universitätsmedizin, Berlin, Germany

At the beginning of this century, the medical faculty at Charité University Medicine Berlin fundamentally revised its curriculum due to the discontentment of its students. However, with the installation of the New Revised Medical Curriculum, the newly created modules appeared unfinished and needed improvement. To address these problems, several students began gathering ideas to aid curricular development. The faculty management later appointed these students as so-called "student module co-directors" (SMCDs).

We have numerous different tasks. Specialist representatives and one SMCD form the board for each module. This group works together to develop the module further. Changes that the board initiates include splitting, shifting, and switching courses, providing teaching material or promoting interprofessional teaching. Aside from the board, SMCDs present introductions into their respective modules to the students, explaining its inner structure and sharing their perspectives. Throughout the module itself, the SMCD acts as a contact person for students' requests and remarks. At the end, students can share their teaching-related opinions and criticism with the SMCD, who presents the given information at a board meeting afterwards and consequently initiates related projects. During the term, all SMCDs meet regularly, discussing modular and non-modular problems in the curriculum and instigating projects to solve them. To better explain my work, I can instance a practical histology course, which students found too long. In a group workshop during our bimonthly SMCD meetings, we discussed the optimal length of these classes. I presented the results at a board meeting, and in consequence, those responsible are developing a concept to split the course.

In my experience, the establishment of SMCDs created a constant impetus on improving our curriculum and, hence, student satisfaction. Moreover, the work as an SMCD constitutes an incomparable opportunity to participate in curriculum development, and I was able to gain much-valued experience through it. Therefore, I can highly recommend establishing workgroups of students like SMCDs to other faculties.

A further example of the co-creation of a curriculum theme – social prescribing – is given as a student case study (Box 7.7).

- *Learning resources:* There has been an increase in recent years in collaboratively created learning resources. For example, interviews with LGBTQIA+ patients about their healthcare experiences to support teaching on LGBTQIA+ health (https://open.ed.ac.uk/lgbt-healthcare-101/).
- *Activities:* Students can also be involved in the development of curriculum-related activity such as student electives or student-selected components.

Issues addressed

Whether the focus is on whole courses, modules, or more specific learning activities, a range of issues may be addressed during curriculum co-creation, drawing on the perspectives of the staff and students. Examples are...

- *Curriculum content:* What should be covered, in what depth, for what purpose and how does this relate to other parts of the curriculum? For example, students may consider the proposed content to be too theoretical and not in keeping with the school's policy of an authentic curriculum where relevance to the practice of medicine is a feature.

Box 7.7 Social prescribing champions

An example of student involvement in co-creation of a curriculum theme by Rania Fernandes, University of Dundee

The Social Prescribing Student Champion Scheme (SPSCS) is an organization that primarily comprises of medical students, dedicated to understanding, researching, and getting involved with social prescribing (SP) in their local communities. "Champions" based at each medical school in the UK are generally tasked with the delivery of informal teaching sessions to their peers, and the formal inclusion of social prescribing teaching within the curriculum. As Scottish Regional Lead for the Scheme, I have enjoyed overseeing the variety in teaching methods adopted by Champions at different universities. Some sessions featured link workers and community navigators, who are the major drivers of SP at a grassroots level. Others invited pharmacists to discuss pharmacological therapies, Numbers Needed to Treat and how community activities could complement medical management.

Personally, this role and the responsibilities that accompany it have changed my outlook and perspective on various aspects of healthcare systems, both locally and abroad. In Portugal, there has been growing enthusiasm among general practitioners to offer medical students the opportunity of observing SP consultations. Locally in Scotland, there are multiple avenues for academic research and creativity. For example, a team of medical students has explored the impact of the COVID-19 pandemic on SP services and how they are delivered. This has led to conversations across a variety of organisations, from the grassroots level to a more legislative degree.

Online modules are a common mode of delivering teaching, and this extends to even foundation doctors. A team of medical students and foundation doctors took the initiative to set up an e-learning module based on SP. This module, hoped to be released later in the year, aims to inform the typical healthcare professional on the aims of SP, the type of patient that is suitable for SP, and how a referral can be made. Besides working on the content of this module, it was a good insight into the more technology-based aspects of e-learning, and the practical, hands-on experience of designing a module was invaluable!

Overall, there are plenty of opportunities to educate fellow medical students and other healthcare professionals. However, most of these are non-funded and require a team of dedicated individuals. With the pressures and time constraints of a medical degree, placements, and other assessments, some student-led projects can often take longer to complete. However, it is a satisfying process once completed and is always an added bonus if it can contribute to your portfolio!

- *Expectations:* What is the expected time commitment from the student, and are these expectations feasible and transparent? Do the expected learning outcomes match the learning experiences offered and the course assessment?
- *Assessment:* How will the students' mastery of the course objectives be assessed and feedback provided?
- *Inclusivity:* Do the learning experiences offered cater to and support the diverse group of students and their individual learning needs? Does the curriculum content support students' equality and diversity competence?

The benefits of co-creation

There are significant advantages to be gained if students and teachers work as part-ners in the production of the curriculum or an element of the curriculum. Even a brief faculty-student collaboration experience collaboration has been shown to have a lasting impact on the students' learning and on the curriculum (Duda and Danielson, 2018). Changes for students included a deepened understanding of the course's subject matter, an appreciation of the importance and centrality of course learning objectives, and an increased desire to engage with their own learning more actively. The benefits for faculty were also highlighted:

> It (curriculum co-creation) proves to be an effective tool for faculty development. It nurtured faculty creativity and pedagogical flexibility. It gave faculty permission to start experimenting in their courses that they only contemplated in the past. Furthermore it opened faculty's eyes to student perspectives, difficulties, and challenges, resulting in new instructional design for strategies such as flipped classroom, active learning methods, and experiential learning. Finally, the research team also observed that this process gave faculty a sense of connectedness to other faculty and allowed them to collectively shoulder the responsibility for understanding and improving student learning (Duda and Danielson, 2018, p. 50).

The benefits to be gained from the co-creation of the curriculum were summarised by Bovill (2020) and Cook-Sather et al. (2014).

- Students feel valued and empowered.
- It develops students' sense of belonging.
- It demonstrates that faculty and students value teaching and learning. Otis and Hammond (2010, p. 40) observed "students often remark that they never realised how much their professors care about their teaching and conversely, faculty frequently comment that they never realised how deeply students care about their learning."
- There is an improved understanding (students and teachers) of the course aims and how these can be achieved in practice. A more authentic curriculum with improvements in the delivery of the teaching and learning programme often results.
- The teacher may develop a greater awareness with regard to the factors to consider and choices that need to be made when planning a curriculum.
- Development of skills in the student, including creativity, assertiveness, negotiation, communication, critical thinking, and team working.
- There is a greater motivation of the student with regard to their three basic psychological needs as a self-determined learner, as described in Chapter 5.
  - *Autonomy* – The student has a measure of control over the curriculum development.
  - *Competence* – A feature of co-creation is the ability of the student to demonstrate their competence in aspects of the curriculum.

- *Relatedness* – Curriculum co-creation is a team activity with the student working closely with teachers and other students.
- Students develop a greater metacognitive awareness of how they and their peers learn. It opens up the learning process to be more transparent.

Challenges to co-creation

Despite the benefits, curriculum co-creation is not without its challenges:

- *Institutional culture:* The strategy may not conform to the institution's culture with regard to student engagement, with a dominant view that teaching is something that is done to students. While individual lecturers may work with or show an interest in working with students as co-creators, the school may be situated at the lower steps of the student participation ladder as described in Chapter 11. It is more likely that partnerships will be effective, and the results of any shared projects impactful, if a co-creation approach is supported and adopted by school managers.
- *Power:* There are several ways in which power relations between students and faculty may be challenging. The traditional hierarchy may be threatened by the alterations of the power dynamic between students and teachers; co-creation may be seen as a risky strategy with doubts as to its success, and so have resistance to its implementation. Even when supported, there may be a gap between the rhetoric and enacted practice of collaboration. Martens et al. (2020) reported teachers' views that a prerequisite for co-creation work is that "teachers should have the final say". This prerequisite sits uneasily with the idea of partnership, highlighting that full partnership, in terms of an equal relationship between staff and students, may be difficult to accept. Students and teachers will bring to any co-creation activity, conscious and unconscious expectations, and modes of working that reflect existing power imbalances between students and faculty. This can limit the extent to which students are meaningfully involved. Bovill (2020) describes how she once facilitated a partnership workshop "where a senior staff member told the student member of their group to order a taxi. Her behaviour could be interpreted in different ways, that the student was spoken to dismissively and treated in this instance as a helper not a partner".
- *Practical constraints:* Co-creation may be supported in principle but considered unrealistic in practice. For example, it may be perceived by staff as taking longer than traditional approaches to curriculum development, and by students as taking time away from their medical studies. As noted above in relation to student representation, without being compensated, financial limitations will prevent some students from contributing time to such work.
- *Inclusivity:* There are concerns that only a small number of students are engaged in curriculum co-creation. While this is not a role that all students may want to participate in, it is important to ensure that all students feel that they have that opportunity and none feel excluded.

This may relate to the point above regarding financial barriers to participation. There may also be more subtle barriers including self-confidence or a feeling of belonging that may discourage some from applying.

- *The costs for students:* While addressing inclusivity is essential, and we can see many benefits in co-creation partnerships as noted above, it is also important to consider the potential negative impact on students. It is often students from minoritized groups who are advocating for change in the curriculum. While it is rewarding when change does occur, this can be a long path and there may be a reluctance to change when institutional structures are challenged. Such co-creation work can come at both an emotional cost and a time/energy cost. When such groups are also reflected in differential attainment, the costs of involvement in co-creation work risk negatively impacting academic work.

Making collaboration work

The following are useful to address the challenges that can arise when implementing curriculum co-creation:

- *Advocate for co-creation:* As prerequisites for co-creation, Martens et al. (2020) note that "Teachers must be open to involve students and create dialogues" and "the organisation must be supportive" (Martens et al., 2020). Where there is limited support for co-creation, it is important to draw on successful examples from within other parts of the university or from other medical schools. It may also be possible to start small, with an achievable co-creation task that will allow staff and students to establish a way that works for them, and the results of such work can be used as evidence of the success of a co-creation approach.
- *Tackle power imbalances:* It is important to consider power explicitly at an early stage in the planning of any co-creation activity, and to provide opportunities for issues to be raised throughout the project. Given that some of these issues may be difficult to discuss, and that there may be differences of opinion, it is essential to discuss how to do this in a way that will foster openness. Kapadia (2021), drawing on their experience as a medical student, suggested the following to address the potential power imbalance between the student and the teacher:
  - Staff engage students as colleagues, with issues raised by students recognised by staff as meriting serious consideration
  - An environment of friendliness and openness is created, breaking down barriers of formality
  - Staff are physically present throughout
  - Students are given the freedom to prioritise tasks and their views are acted on and respected
  - Students are consulted on all matters regardless of whether they are small or large
  - Students are encouraged verbally and reassured that their opinion is valued

- *Be realistic about time:* Consider the amount of time that is required (from staff and students) for the intended co-creation work, and where possible, seek funds to pay students for the time spent. If co-creation activities involve a larger group, perhaps the whole class, time should be factored into their normal student hours rather than being added on as an extra commitment. This will also help to level the playing field and ensure that those students with other responsibilities, including caring or part-time work, are not excluded from involvement in co-creation work.
- *Ensure inclusivity:* Ensuring adequate time and/or payment may address some barriers to student involvement, but it is important to consider inclusivity more broadly. Some questions to consider are: How are students selected for involvement, and does this process favour or disadvantage any groups of students? Would the organisation of the work be a barrier to some students? How diverse are the staff involved in co-creation activities, and what impact might this have on student involvement?
- *Provide training:* Both students and teachers should be offered opportunities to develop an understanding of what co-creation involves, what skills are needed, the challenges that may arise and how these may be addressed. Furthermore, there is a need to help students acquire an understanding of, and skills related to, medical education that will support them in their role as co-creator or curriculum collaborator more widely. Many schools now offer training in education as part of the formal undergraduate curriculum, as an elective, or as an intercalated degree course. The twelve-week online AMEE-ESME course for students leads to the award of an AMEE-ESME Certificate in Medical Education. The International Federation of Medical Student Associations has also supported student engagement in curriculum development, including the provision of a toolkit to support student engagement in the improvement of Interprofessional Medical Education. While general training in medical education is valuable, specific training in co-creation is also essential.

Box 7.8 describes the practical steps taken to implement student curriculum co-creation at one university.

Box 7.8 The curriculum student co-creation process implemented at Creighton University, Nebraska

From *Duda, G.K., Danielson, M.A., 2018. Collaborative curricular (re)construction— tracking faculty and student learning impacts and outcomes five years later. Int. J. Stud. Partners. 2 (2), 39–52.*

- One or more faculty members are asked to identify a course that would benefit from redesign and student input
- A student is recruited who has taken the course recently
- Faculty and student meet at least six times individually and in working groups over several months, culminating in a large-group meeting. Small groups may meet weekly
- Faculty and student each receive an educational text and the equivalent of $100

Conclusion

The student as a curriculum collaborator is at the forefront of the agenda with regard to student engagement with the education programme. The student as an evaluator of teaching and learning and as a member of the curriculum committee is now widely, if not universally, accepted. The student as a co-creator of the curriculum is gaining ground, and the benefits that result from student and staff working closely together in curriculum co-creation are now well established. Close attention should be given to the form that staff-student partnership working takes to ensure that both students' and staff expectations are met and that the work enhances the curriculum.

References

Alfonso, N.M., Cardozo, L.J., Mascarenhas, O.A.J., Aranha, A.N.F., Shah, C., 2005. Are anonymous evaluations a better assessment of faculty teaching performance? A comparative analysis of open and anonymous evaluation processes. Fam. Med. 37 (1), 43–47.

Berk, R.A., 2013. Top five flashpoints in the assessment of teaching effectiveness. Med. Teach. 35 (1), 15–26.

Behrend, R., Franz, A., Czeskleba, A., Maaz, A., Peters, H., 2019. Student participation in the development of interprofessional education courses: Perceptions and experiences of faculty members and the students. Med. Teach. 41 (12), 1366–1371.

Boomer, G., Lester, N., Onore, C., Cook, J., 1992. Negotiating the curriculum: Educating for the 21st century. Falmer Press, London, UK.

Bovill, C., 2013. Students and staff co-creating curricula: A new trend or an old idea we never got around to implementing? In: Rust, C. (Ed.), Improving Student Learning Through Research and Scholarship: 20 Years of ISL. Oxford Centre for Staff and Learning Development, Oxford, UK.

Bovill, C., 2020. Co-creation in learning and teaching: The case for a whole-class approach in higher education. High. Educ. 79, 1023–1037.

Bovill, C., Cook-Sather, A., Felten, P., Millard, L., Moore-Cherry, N., 2016. Addressing potential challenges in co-creating learning and teaching: Overcoming resistance, navigating institutional norms and ensuring inclusivity in student–staff partnerships. High. Educ. 71 (2), 195–208.

Bron, J., Bovill, C., Veugelers, W., 2016. Students experiencing and developing democratic citizenship through curriculum negotiation: The relevance of Garth Boomer's approach. Curric. Persp. 36 (1), 15–27.

Bryson, C., 2014. Understanding and Developing Student Engagement. Routledge, London, UK.

Cook-Sather, A., Bovill, C., Felten, P., 2014. Engaging Students as Partners in Learning and Teaching: A Guide for Faculty. Jossey-Bass, San Francisco, USA.

Crawford, K., 2012. Rethinking the student/teacher nexus: Students as consultants on teaching in higher education. In: Neary, M., Bell, L., Stevenson, H. (Eds.), Towards Teaching in Public: Reshaping the Modern University. Continuum, London, UK.

Duda, G.K., Danielson, M.A., 2018. Collaborative curricular (re)construction—tracking faculty and student learning impacts and outcomes five years later. Int. J. Stud. Partners. 2 (2), 39–52.

Englander, R., Holmboe, E., Batalden, P., Caron, R.M., Durham, C.F., Foster, T., Ogrinc, G., Ercan-Fang, N., Batalden, M., 2020. Coproducing health professions education: A prerequisite to coproducing health care services? Acad. Med. 95 (7), 1006–1013.

Fan, Y., Shepherd, L.J., Slavich, E., Waters, D., Stone, M., Abel, R., Johnston, E.L., 2019. Gender and cultural bias in student evaluations: Why representation matters. PLOS ONE. 14 (2), e0209749.

Freyd, M., 1923. The Graphic Rating Scale. J. Educ. Psychol. 14 (2), 83–102.

Harden, J., Fawkner, S., 2019. A student partnership project to enhance curriculum development in medical education [Blog post, January 24th]. Teaching Matters Blog. Accessed at: http://www.teaching-matters-blog.ed.ac.uk/a-student-partnership-project-to-enhance-curriculum-development-in-medical-education/.

Heffernan, T., 2022. Sexism, racism, prejudice, and bias: A literature review and synthesis of research surrounding student evaluations of courses and teaching. Assess. Eval. High. Educ. 47 (1), 144–154.

Hessler, M., Pöpping, D.M., Hollstein, H., Ohlenburg, H., Arnemann, P.H., Massoth, C., Seidel, L.M., Zarbock, A., Wenk, M., 2018. Availability of cookies during an academic course session affects evaluation of teaching. Med. Educ. 52 (10), 1064–1072.

Kapadia, S.J., 2021. Perspectives of a 2nd-year medical student on 'Students as Partners' in higher education - What are the benefits, and how can we manage the power dynamics? Med. Teach. 43 (4), 478–479.

Könings, K.D., Mordang, S., Smeenk, F., Stassen, L., Ramani, S., 2021. Learner involvement in the co-creation of teaching and learning: AMEE Guide No. 138. Med. Teach. 43 (8), 924–936.

Kumar, P., Pickering, C.M., Atta, L., Burns, A.G., Chu, R.F., Gracie, T., Qin, C.X., Whang, K.A., Goldberg, H.R., 2020. Student curriculum review team, 8 years later: Where we stand and opportunities for growth. Med. Teach. 43 (3), 314–319.

Little, B., Locke, W., Scesa, A., Williams, R., 2009. Report to HEFCE on Student Engagement. Higher Education Funding Council for England, Bristol, UK.

MacNell, L., Driscoll, A., Hunt, A., 2015. What's in a name: exposing gender bias in student ratings of teaching. Innov. High. Educ. 40 (4), 291–303.

Martens, S.E., Wolfhagen, I.H.A.P., Whittingham, J.R.D., Dolmans, D.H.J.M., 2020. Mind the gap: Teachers' concep-

tions of student-staff partnership and its potential to enhance educational quality. Med. Teach. 42 (5), 529–535.

Mitchell, K., Martin, J., 2018. Gender bias in student evaluations. PS. Polit. Sci. Polit. 51 (3), 648–652.

Otis, M.M., Hammond, J.D., 2010. Participatory action research as a rationale for student voices in the scholarship of teaching and learning. In: Werder, C., Otis, M.M. (Eds.), Engaging Student Voices in the Study of Teaching and Learning. Stylus Publishing, Sterling, Virginia, USA.

Peterson, D.A.M., Biederman, L.A., Andersen, D., Ditonto, T.M., Roe, K., 2019. Mitigating gender bias in student evaluations of teaching. PLOS ONE. 14 (5), e0216241.

Ryan, M., 2015. Framing student evaluations of university learning and teaching: discursive strategies and textual outcomes. Assess. Eval. High. Educ. 40 (8), 1142–1158.

Schiekirka, S., Feufel, M.A., Herrmann-Lingen, C., Raupach, T., 2015. Evaluation in medical education: A topical review of target parameters, data collection tools and confounding factors. Ger. Med. Sci. 13, Doc15.

Scott, K.W., Callahan, D.G., Chen, J.J., et al., 2019. Fostering student–faculty partnerships for continuous curricular improvement in undergraduate medical education. Acad. Med. 94 (7), 996–1001.

Steyer, T.E., Ravenell, R.L., Mainous, A.G., Blue, A.V., 2003. The role of medical students in curriculum committees. Teach. Learn. Med. 15 (4), 238–241.

Stukalina, Y., 2014. Identifying predictors of student satisfaction and student motivation in the framework of assuring quality in the delivery of higher education services. Bus. Man. Educ. 12 (1), 127–137.

Tang, W., Jianning, B., Liu, J., Wang, H., Chen, Q., 2012. Students' evaluation indicators of the curriculum. Int. J. Med. Educ. 3, 103–106.

Tucker, B., 2014. Student evaluation surveys: anonymous comments that offend or are unprofessional. High. Educ. 68 (3), 347–358.

The student as an assessor | 8

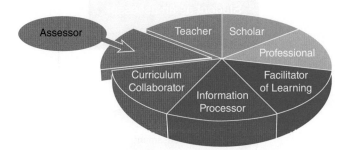

Sharing responsibility for assessment

Assessment is important to the maintenance of standards and to the legitimacy of the degree and institution. Key questions that should be asked about assessment include why assess?, how to assess?, when to assess?, what to assess?, and who does the assessing? (Falchikov, 2005; Harden and Laidlaw, 2021). The answer to the question of "who" includes the teacher or school assessment committee; accrediting bodies; employers; the patient; and, importantly, students themselves. The student as an actor has a valuable role to play in the medical school in the assessment process.

In this chapter, we look at the benefits to be gained from examining the assessment process through the student lens, bringing to bear the student's perspective on assessment decisions. We then explore two areas where the student has a unique role to play – peer assessment and self-assessment (Figure 8.1). In both of these areas, students can make a valuable contribution to assessment decisions beyond that which can be offered by the teacher.

While there has been a move to engage students in the planning and delivery of the curriculum, as described in Chapter 7, student involvement in assessment decisions remains less common. Student evaluation is often a decision made by teachers with little or no consultation with students. Beaman (1998, p. 48) gives an example of the problem outside higher education.

> *A manager walks in one morning and tells his staff 'I have completed some training that explains the power and promise of individual empowerment. Starting today you will be allowed to manage your own time schedules,*

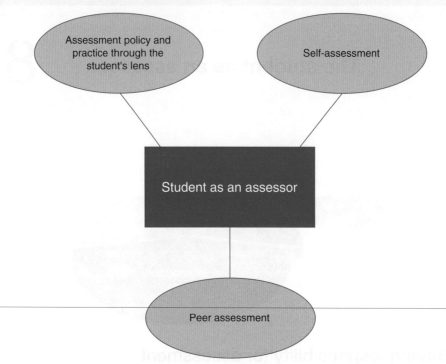

Figure 8.1 The student's role as an assessor.

create your own work teams, design your own work space, and manage daily organisational responsibilities. YOU ARE EMPOWERED! Then, at the end of each week, I will be evaluating you on criteria that I will set and measure... just to make sure everything is working out fine. Thank you and good luck'.

This example highlights the significance of power in assessment. Indeed, it was pointed out by Reynolds and Trehan (2000) that

More than any other aspect of education, assessment embodies power relations between the institution and its students, with tutors as custodians of the institution's rules and practices...while there are some examples of critical pedagogy affecting content and method, corresponding changes in the practice of assessment are harder to find.

Heron (1981) warned that

Assessment is the most political of all educational processes, it is where issues of power are most at stake. If there is no staff/student collaboration in assessment then staff exert a stranglehold that inhibits the development of collaboration with respect to all other processes.

There may seem to be inherent contradictions in relation to students as the object of assessment and student engagement with the determination of assessment policy and practice. However, just as the student can bring a valuable perspective to decisions about the curriculum, so too the student can make a valuable contribution to the school's assessment policy and practice.

The Quality Assurance Agency (2018a), has argued for the sharing of responsibility for assessment. Dialogue with students helps to develop student confidence that assessment is designed to be inclusive, allows for reasonable adjustments in individual cases where necessary, and is fair and consistent (2018b). Addressing the benefits of student involvement, Falchikov (2005) argued that

> Involving students in assessment has the power to redress many of the negative aspects of traditional teacher led assessment and student involvement is a means to improve the quality of assessment rather than acting as a barrier to it.

Portnoy (2019) highlighted the benefits for students:

> When educators share the responsibility of assessment with their students, students become more self-reflective, independent learners who achieve greater agency and voice within the classroom.

Terms used to indicate this sharing of responsibility by students and teachers for assessment include *collaborative assessment, co-assessment,* and *participative assessment.* (Falchikov, 2005).

Assessment through the student lens

Harden and Lilley (2018) describe ten steps in the implementation of a school's assessment programme (Box 8.1). The student's voice and perspective can contribute to the steps in the process.

Steps 1-3: Students can engage in discussions related to the approach to assessment and application of the criteria for good assessment. They can contribute their perspectives as to where the school currently lies on each of the dimensions in a school's *"Assessment PROFILE"* and where a school *should* be with regard to its assessment policies and practices (Harden and Lilley, 2018) (Figure 8.2). Such a discussion could contribute to the agreement about a consensus policy regarding a school's future policy in relation to assessment.

Students should also be able to give their views as to whether the assessment process in the medical school corresponds to the criteria for good assessment (individual and systems) as described in the Ottawa Consensus Report on the subject (Norcini et al., 2011; 2018). The different criteria may not apply equally in all assessments and in all situations, but the student's perspective on their application in the context of the medical school will be helpful in the quality enhancement of assessments.

Step 4: Students can be involved in ensuring that communication about assessments is adequate. It is good practice to ask students to review assessment instructions or guidance, to ensure that the expectations are clear. It is important to

Box 8.1 Ten steps in a school's assessment programme (Harden and Lilley, 2018)

1. Decisions are made on the institution's overall approach to assessment in relation to the issues identified in the school's Assessment PROFILE.
2. The overall timing and form of examinations, the learning outcomes assessed, the tools to be used and the staff responsible are determined.
3. Individual assessments such as an OSCE or written examination are developed, and the learning outcomes assessed are specified.
4. The students are briefed about the examination, including its form, areas covered and the implications for their progress.
5. The resources for the examination are prepared. This will vary depending on whether it is paper-based, computer-based, or clinical.
6. The examination is implemented, and evidence about the students' performance is collected.
7. Based on the evidence obtained from this and other assessments, decisions are made about the individual student as to whether they have reached the standard required.
8. Feedback is provided to students about their performance in the examination.
9. Feedback is also provided to examiners and teachers.
10. The examination process is reviewed.

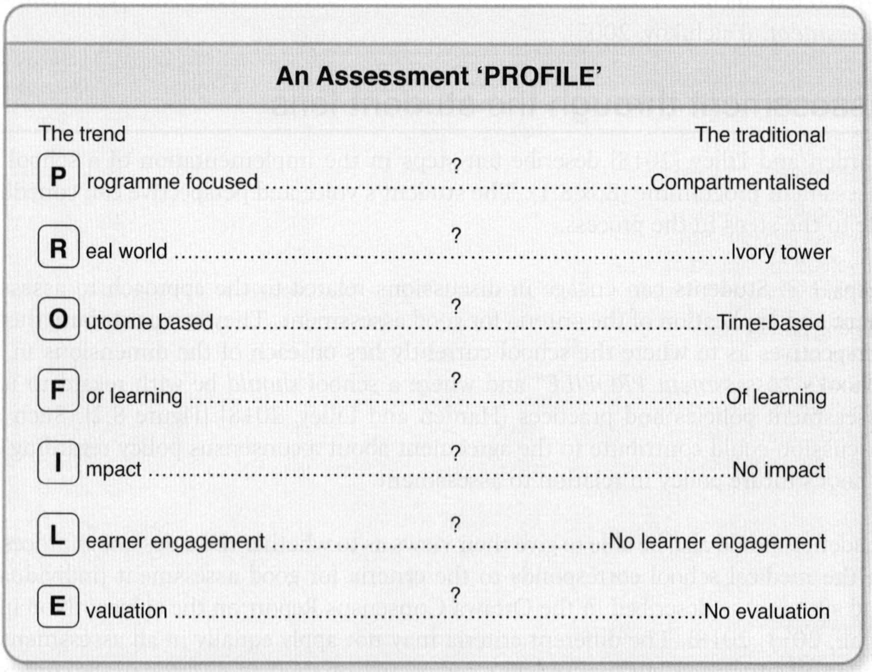

An Assessment 'PROFILE'

The trend		The traditional
P rogramme focused	?	Compartmentalised
R eal world	?	Ivory tower
O utcome based	?	Time-based
F or learning	?	Of learning
I mpact	?	No impact
L earner engagement	?	No learner engagement
E valuation	?	No evaluation

Figure 8.2 The seven *Assessment PROFILE* dimensions with the end anchor points identified in each dimension (Harden and Lilley, 2018).

Students can contribute to a discussion as to where the school should lie on each dimension.

identify ways to enhance students' assessment literacy; their knowledge, skills, and understanding of the assessment process (Rhind et al., 2021). Rhind et al. conducted workshops with veterinary medical students to give them experience in the standard setting process. The students reported that this experience enhanced their understanding of the process. For example, one said

> *Interesting! Didn't realize as much work went into checking the questions were at the right level. Makes me feel more confident about the process in general. Good to understand how it all works (p. 159).*

Step 5: Most assessments will be "unseen": so to preserve the integrity of the assessment there are limits to students' involvement in preparing such assessments. While it may be possible to involve senior students in preparing exams for earlier year groups, this would place considerable trust in the students not to share any questions. Where assessments are made available to students in advance (for example, an essay), students can be involved in the development of the assessment, criteria, and guidance for students.

Step 6: It may be possible to consider involving senior students as examiners for clinical examinations among earlier years: this encourages schools to consider the required expertise of examiners. Students can be involved also in OSCEs as simulated patients. In Box 8.2, we present reflections from a student on their experience as a simulated patient.

Box 8.2 Student case study: the student as a simulated patient

Reflections on the experience of being a simulated patient, by Emily Burns, University of Edinburgh

During the 3rd year of my medical degree, I had the opportunity to be a Simulated Patient for the Objective Structured Clinical Examinations (OSCEs) for the earlier year groups. This involved me acting as a patient so that the students could perform certain examinations or take a history from me, all whilst being assessed by an examiner.

Taking part in this gave me a key insight into the OSCE which I had not experienced before. I had previously taken part in these clinical examinations as a student being assessed, so it was very interesting for me to see it from a different point of view. It also allowed me to chat with the examiners and ask them what they look for when assessing students. One of the common critiques that cropped up several times was the student's interactions with simulated patients. Each examiner expressed to me the importance of good communication skills and that they are just as, if not more important, as the clinical skills themselves.

I gained a lot from this experience, and it has benefitted my clinical practice tremendously. Being able to experience the OSCE as a patient has allowed me to further appreciate the importance of good communication and people skills. I have taken what I have learned from this experience and incorporated it into my own practice. As a result, one of the main pieces of positive feedback I receive from my consultations is that I am very good at interacting with patients.

I would strongly encourage every student to take part in something like this as it allows you to develop well-rounded consultation skills. If you are unable to do that, there are ways you can acquire similar skills through speaking to patients whilst on placement. You can ask patients about their positive and negative experiences in previous consultations and learn from them.

Step 7: It is unlikely that students will be involved in any decisions made about individual performance, unless they are, as noted in Step 6, also examiners.

Step 8: Students can be involved in discussions around how and when feedback on performance is given, immediately after the examination or at a later date, and individually or in groups.

Steps 9-10: Students can evaluate the assessment process. Their feedback can be gathered through the end-of-course/module questionnaires or via student representatives.

Consideration should be given to the ways in which students can be meaningfully involved. As with curriculum committees, as discussed in Chapter 7, students can and should be involved in assessment committees. Where this is not current practice, it may be useful to consult with students as to how best to include them in the management structures related to assessment processes. Where students are already represented on the committee, it is good practice to offer them the opportunity to review their involvement and reflect on what works and what might be improved.

While much of the focus of student involvement in assessment is on the process, it is also useful to connect the student's role as curriculum collaborator with their role as assessor. Greenstein and Burke (2020) emphasised that student engagement in assessment includes "asking students for their input on what should be measured". These are potentially challenging questions about who decides what answers are "correct" or what performance constitutes an acceptable demonstration of competency. While in some areas there may be little doubt or debate, there are other areas where there is uncertainty; for example, empathy is not a clear or definitive category to assess, and the criteria for demonstrating empathy are not standardised. As such, it is one example where it would be useful to engage the students in developing the curriculum (how empathy is defined; how/where in the curriculum it is taught; and how it is assessed).

Peer assessment

Much of the attention paid to student engagement with the assessment process has been directed at peer assessment. In peer assessment, the student applies agreed-upon standards to critique the work of other learners and makes decisions or offers feedback about it.

> Peer assessment involves taking responsibility for assessing the work of their peers against set assessment criteria. It's a powerful way for your student to act as the 'assessor' and to gain a better understanding of assessment criteria. It can also transfer some ownership of the assessment process to them, thereby potentially increasing their motivations and engagements (University of Reading, 2021).

Peer assessment as an aid to learning

Peer assessment, if incorporated into the education programme, can serve as an aid to learning. Students may be asked to evaluate the work of their colleagues, and at the same time provide constructive feedback relating to areas of potential improvement and recommended further study. Here are some examples of the use of peer assessment used to improve learning:

- Students organise a mock OSCE to prepare their colleagues for the formal examination and evaluate their colleague's performance, providing feedback about the performance. In Box 8.3, we present a student's experiences of being involved in the development of mock OSCEs.
- Students evaluate and provide feedback with regard to presentations or assignments prepared by their colleagues
- Students write MCQs for their peers. For example, the PeerWise system enables students to author questions, answer and rate their peers' questions, and provide comments. Through this approach, students can actively engage in peer assessment and gain insight into the question setting from an examiner's perspective.

In these situations, peer assessment is often formative. Peer assessment can also be used summatively. The involvement of students as assessors for summative assessments, however, is more challenging with built-in safeguards required, which we discuss below.

Box 8.3   Student case study: peer-peer mock OSCEs

An example of student-led mock OSCE revision sessions, by Helena Martin, University of Edinburgh

Shortly after we were informed that the first OSCEs of our clinical years would be held virtually because of the COVID-19 pandemic, I organised a series of virtual OSCE revision sessions. The OSCE revision sessions involved 8 individual Zoom rooms with 8 students and 2 assessor-actors. Each student took the lead on one station before receiving personal feedback and formalised mark-scheme feedback (2 minutes).

Peers enjoyed the novel format of the sessions whereby the 7 non-performing students were able to listen to their peer's OSCE performance. This could pose as both peer-to-peer passive learning and active learning during their one OSCE station performance where they received personalised tutor-actor feedback. Of course, this relied on students staying focussed in their 7 non-performing stations – which is arguably the biggest challenge in online teaching. Additionally, leading an 8-minute OSCE station under the scrutiny of 7 peers would probably not be seen as appropriate if the session had been organised by more senior tutors or the medical school itself. Perhaps we have found a niche for peer-to-peer teaching that formal teaching cannot satisfy.

When developing the mock OSCEs, my "imposter syndrome" was roaring as I had only completed 8 summative OSCE sessions in my medical school career thus far. However, the sessions were an overall success. On obtaining feedback from participants, I discovered the written feedback followed the "polite peer paradox" – whereby improvements were very polite, and no blame was placed on any individual organiser or tutor. Instead, feedback was either "N/A – it was really useful" or noted technical difficulties as the only problem. Polite feedback is confidence-building but likely held back the pace of improvements in our OSCE revision sessions. It was only until I received social media messages from closer friends who had attended and when I quizzed friends after the sessions, I could really reflect on the successes of the sessions in being appropriately "scary".

The use of peer assessment as a measure of a student's professionalism and attitudes

The assessment of a student's professionalism and their attitude to patients in practice is important and should be part of the final assessment of a student prior to graduation. However, this presents challenges not represented by the assessment of other learning outcomes using traditional assessment methods. Triangulation from a range of sources, including 360-degree feedback, is required. Compared to the teacher, fellow students, with their more intimate knowledge of a colleague's attitudes and behaviour, are in a good, perhaps even a better position to make a judgement (Box 8.4). Nevertheless, the personal knowledge that students may have of each other can also pose challenges for peer assessment, which we discuss below.

Peer assessment of a student's contribution to group work

The assessment of an individual student's contribution to a group task can be challenging. Peer assessment can provide a more accurate picture of the individual's performance and contribution to group work (Cheng and Warren, 2000). It is recognised that students may not contribute equally when engaged in a group task, with some students "free riding". There may be individual differences in contributions to the group task, commitment to the task, following agreed-upon rules for the group work, management of areas of conflict, and time prioritisation.

A score or grade may be awarded to a group for its work. The same score can be awarded to all members of the group, but it may be fairer if scores are awarded to individual group members based on their contribution to the group (McIntyre and Crawford, 2022). Members of the group can reach an agreement about the contributions other group members have made. Falchikov (2005, Chapter 9) reviews different approaches to redistributing the group score to the individual members of the group:

- Splitting the group mark between group members
- Multiplication of the group mark by an individual weighting factor
- Using the group mark plus or minus a minor individual contribution mark
- Sharing equally the group mark with exceptional tutor interventions
- The use of yellow or red cards with individuals given a yellow card having a percentage reduction of the group mark and a red card attracting a zero grade

---

Box 8.4 The case of Harold Shipman

Harold Shipman, a General Practitioner in the UK, was found guilty of being responsible for the deaths of more than 300 of his patients as a result of his inappropriate behaviour as a doctor. A colleague of Shipman's from medical school confided in me (RMH), that this came as no surprise to her. As a medical student, he had demonstrated inappropriate behaviour and attitudes toward patients. This problem was recognised by other students but was not identified in the school's formal examinations, and he qualified from medical school having passed the necessary examinations. Peer assessment may have identified the problem.

Advantages of peer assessment

A number of benefits may be gained from engaging students in peer assessment.

> *Peer assessment is a natural extension of the move from a teacher-centred to a student-centred model of education, which emphasises the active engagement of students in their learning, learning responsibility, metacognitive skills, and dialogical, collaborative model of teaching and learning (Wride, 2017).*

Peer assessment:

- Motivates students by giving them a sense of ownership of the assessment process
- Gives students an insight into the curriculum, including the expected learning outcomes and an understanding of the assessment process
- Emphasises that assessment is part of learning
- Encourages collaborative learning
- Recognises teamwork skills are an important learning outcome of the education programme
- Prepares students for a peer assessment role when later they are practising members of a healthcare team. This is a feature of continuing professional development and is a UK General Medical Council (GMC) requirement
- Provides a valid assessment of a student's professionalism and contribution to group work

Challenges associated with peer assessment

Falchikov (2005) explores common problems associated with peer assessment and their possible solutions.

- *Responsibility for assessment:* Teachers and students may see assessment as the teacher's responsibility. Falchikov (p. 151) notes that teachers often ask, "Isn't it my job as a teacher to undertake assessment?" and that those who ask this question "may have difficulty in changing their role in response to current ideas about student-centred learning and teaching". Students may feel that involvement with peer assessment takes time away from their studies and that it should be the teacher's responsibility. It is important therefore to explain the benefits of peer assessment to both teachers and students. Teachers can also be reassured that they still have an important role to play in training students in their assessment role and monitoring their work as an assessor.
- *Potential for bias:* Students and staff may be concerned that bias will affect peer assessment. Students often know each in personal contexts which may influence their assessment of peers, particularly when assessing something more fluid, such as professionalism. For example, if a peer says or does something at a party that shows they might have misogynistic views, this may influence a peer assessment of professionalism, even if no such views were demonstrated in the educational setting. The insight that students have of each other can be an advantage of peer assessment, but it is not

straightforward to apply and requires explicit discussion of difficult instances, such as the example given, to help students perform peer assessments fairly and with integrity. Studies have shown that with the necessary training, satisfactory reliability in terms of the agreement between the tutor and peer marks can be found.

Bias of this kind is not inevitable; rather it is seen to be an outcome of some breakdown in commitment, understanding, or trust by students engaged in rating their peers (Magin, 2001, p. 62).

Bias may be less of a problem when students are rated, not just by one other student, but by all members of a group with the peer mark determined by averaging the ratings of the students. This can compensate for differences in ratings or standards in the same way that OSCE variations in examiners' standards are compensated for with the use of a number of examiners. Assessment can be seen as the collective decision made by a group of students, and a justification may also be required to defend a rating. It is also important to have a clear complaints process so that students are aware of how to raise a concern and how this will be dealt with. Some thought should be given to who would be involved in this process and how to involve students as well as faculty to ensure that all students feel comfortable making complaints and confident that their concerns will be taken seriously.

- *Impact on relationships:* Students often feel uncomfortable assessing the competence of their colleagues and may be concerned that peer assessment, particularly with the award of low scores, will have an impact on their immediate relationships with peers and also future relationships with them as colleagues. It may be useful to include experiences of such concerns from senior students or junior doctors to demonstrate that these concerns are common but mostly unfounded. It is also important to remind students of the support processes in the school to ensure that they feel supported should any issues arise.
- *Competency as assessors:* Students may lack confidence in their ability to assess each other in a fair and responsible way. This can be tackled if training and support are provided. With practice and experience, students become more confident. In Box 8.5, we present a student case study that discusses a peer observation of a teaching scheme including the training of peer assessors.

Implementation

If peer assessment is adopted, attention should be paid to its implementation. This should be carefully planned and monitored, with training provided for students.

- Monitoring of peer assessment by staff is particularly important if the assessment is used for summative processes. In this case, it should be possible for the peer assessment grades awarded by students to be adjusted where necessary and any unfair or inappropriate marking dealt with. Peer marking should be carried out in a classroom situation under examination conditions to prevent collusion between students.
- The expected learning outcomes or competencies against which a student is to be assessed must be made explicit. The peer assessor should understand

> **Box 8.5** Student case study: assessing teaching competence - peer observation of teaching
>
> *An example of a student-led peer observation of teaching scheme, by Ed Whittaker, University of Edinburgh*
>
> A group of students at Edinburgh Medical School, including myself, are passionate about near-peer teaching. In our group's experience, for years, "assessment" of teaching consisted of a rushed google form as people put on their coats to leave, with generic questions and equally generic answers, with low response rates and little focus on our teaching skills. We thought we could do something more beneficial for our teaching development and set up a Peer Observation of Teaching (POT) programme.
>
> We were trained on the approaches of providing feedback, and using a previously developed model we observed near-peer medical teaching sessions, with a pre- and post-observation meeting. We assessed the observees' planning, delivery, and any specific concerns regarding their teaching, providing verbal and written feedback.
>
> Research we carried out after the peer teaching observations, comprising surveys and focus groups, suggested that both undergraduate peer assessors and observees can gain from the experience of POT. Observees found feedback valuable, learning about, reflecting on, and increasing confidence in teaching practice. They felt comfortable receiving feedback and reported positively about the observers in terms of expertise, relatability, non-intimidating presence, and awareness of the target audience. Assessors also said that they found the experience of observing others and providing feedback a useful learning experience, but many also said that they lacked confidence in their credibility. For example, one said "I don't know more what I'm talking about than them. I feel like maybe I didn't make it peer-y enough. I think my session may have turned into more like me acting. So, I don't know if that's just imposter syndrome".
>
> I suggest that further work should analyse how best to implement POT into the medical curriculum and to improve teaching practice in medical students by normalising its use, and further training and/or coaching could be considered to overcome assessors' perceived barriers to POT. Ultimately, I believe as peers we have a lot of experiences to share with each other, and I hope through peer assessment and collaborative discussions, my own and others' peer teaching practices will continue to benefit.

what success and mastery looks like to allow them to assess how near their colleague has come to achieving this. Rubrics or checklists against which the student can be assessed can be provided to facilitate the assessment. Checklists are commonly used in the OSCE to guide less experienced examiners.

- Training for students should include the rationale for utilising peer assessment; the process of undertaking peer assessment; and opportunities to try peer assessment, initially in simulated situations. The psychometric properties of peer assessment are improved by the training of peer assessors and their further experience (Zundert et al., 2010). Two examples of games that can be used as part of the training are given in Box 8.6. The co-creation of the training programme with students is likely to enhance its efficacy.

Self-assessment

When considering the role of the student in assessment, the assessment by students of their own achievements is important. Self-assessment is the descriptive and evaluative act carried out by the student concerning their own work and academic abilities (Brown and Harris, 2013). Self-assessment overlaps with the

> **Box 8.6** Two examples of games used in training programmes
>
> **The Egg Game for introducing students to peer assessment (Beaman 1998, p. 53)**
>
> Groups of five or six students are asked to make an egg container that can be dropped from a certain height without the eggs breaking. Each group prepares the criteria on which they will assess both the process and the product. They determine how much weighting or what percentage to be allocated to each criterion.
>
> **"You can get a raise" exercise for assessing contributions to group work (Beaman 1998, p. 54)**
>
> Each group of students is given $1000 in Monopoly money for doing a good job on a project or whatever is going on at the time. They are asked to divide the money among group members according to the amount and quality of work they contributed to the bonus. The doling out or withholding of monopoly money was found better than verbal or written evaluations.

concepts of self-evaluation, self-appraisal, and self-reflection, which apply to the individual looking reflectively at their own work and assessing their own abilities against a set of standards. Critical self-appraisal is the hallmark of a good professional. Costa and Kallick (1992) suggest that

> *We must constantly remind ourselves that the ultimate purpose of evaluation is to have students become self-evaluating. If students graduate from our schools still dependent upon others to tell them when they are adequate, good or excellent, then we've missed the whole point of what education is about.*

Why self-assessment

Experience with self-assessment should be an important component of the undergraduate medical curriculum, and there is widespread advocacy for self-assessment as a powerful learning process for a number of reasons:

- *Self-assessment is an important part of the learning process.* It allows the learner to diagnose their own learning needs and to take the necessary action to meet these.

  From a pedagogical perspective, effective learning can only occur when students have a realistic sense of their own performance so that they can direct their further learning on the critical aspects of their learning needs (Yan et al., 2020).

- Self-assessment has been extensively recommended as an appropriate approach to student involvement in assessment as part of wider support for "assessment for learning". Through the practice of self-assessment, students are encouraged to reflect on what they have learned, to integrate new knowledge with their existing knowledge base, to make more effective use of learning resources, and to develop themselves as self-regulated learners. Self-assessment, therefore, plays a vital role in students' involvement in the roles described in Chapters 5 and 6.
- *Improved academic performance:* The engagement with learning that results from self-assessment has a positive effect on academic performance (Zimmerman and Schunke, 2011).

A logical explanation of the positive relationship between self-assessment and learning gains is that engagement in self-assessment practices may encourage students to seek feedback and reflect on their own performance which in turn lead to improved learning (Yan 2018, p. 184).

- *Career development:* Self-assessment is a feature of the continuing professional development that a doctor should engage in throughout life as a medical practitioner. The medical course should prepare the student to assess their own competence as one of the core skills necessary for life-long learning.

Even excellent doctors can develop bad habits and become outdated. These will show up in the mirror of self-assessment (Harden and Laidlaw, 1992).

While used for the most part formatively, in specific contexts self-assessment can be used for summative purposes. While there are some concerns that self-assessment may generate inaccurate assessment results, with poor students overestimating their achievements and good students underestimating their achievements (Eva and Regehr, 2008), these can be overcome through guidance and experience with self-assessment. It is also important to set realistic, specific self-assessment opportunities. Task-specific assessments, such as the assessment of communication skills in a station in an OSCE, may be more helpful than a global assessment of communication skills. Eva and Regehr (2008) noted

We suspect most people are prompted to open a dictionary as a result of encountering a word for which they are uncertain of the meaning rather than out of a broader assessment that their vocabulary could be improved (p. 16).

Training in self-assessment

Self-assessment is not an innate skill; it is a habit that needs to be acquired by students (Box 8.7). Self-assessment should be recognised not as a single event but as a cyclical process in which self-assessment judgements are gradually refined. Experiences gained in self-assessment increase students' familiarity with the process and build confidence in the learners' capacity to realistically assess their own achievements.

Students need to have multiple opportunities to develop the skill of realistically evaluating their own work so that they can gain confidence in their capacity, therefore self-assessment activity should be regarded as routine in learning and instruction so that students have opportunity to engage in veridical or realistic self-assessment (Yan et al., 2020).

Box 8.7   Self-assessment skills have to be learned

Following a written examination students were given the opportunity in a lecture theatre to mark their own paper based on a model answer and a rubric provided. To my surprise (RMH), faced with the task of identifying the deficiencies in their answers three students became highly disturbed and were unable to complete the exercise. This was the first time that they had the experience of assessing themselves in this way. They needed better preparation for the task and more experience with self-assessment.

While practice is important on its own, it is insufficient to improve self-assessment abilities. Skills in self-assessment should be formally taught (Brown and Harris, 2014), and further work needs to be done to establish how these skills might be best taught (Yan and Brown, 2017). The different actions undertaken in self-assessment should be explored with students to help them in their role as self-assessors and to enhance the accuracy of self-assessment (Brown et al., 2015):

- Clarification of the assessment criteria
- Self-directed feedback seeking
- Self-reflection

Clarification of the assessment criteria

Before students can assess themselves, they must understand the standards or criteria against which they will be judged. O'Donovan et al. (2008, p. 215) described the different positions with regard to students' understanding of assessment standards:

- *A laissez-faire approach* with standards communicated informally and serendipitously. This was common in the past in medical education.
- *An explicit statement of what is expected* with the adoption of outcome-based/competency-based education. This is now standard practice. For example, in an OSCE, the checklist for a station may provide the criteria against which the student can judge themselves. However, the expected standards may not be clearly referred to or understood by students.
- *Engagement of learners* in using the standards and applying them in a situation. Earlier in the chapter, we noted the example of running standard setting workshops for students, to facilitate their understanding of this part of the assessment process (Rhind et al., 2021). In addition to this, it can also be useful to create opportunities for students to work in small groups and mark exemplar assignments. Where appropriate to the assessment, video demonstrations of a procedure which is the subject of a self-assessment may serve as an example of what is expected and the standard required. In a study described by Hawkins et al. (2012), students were shown a video recording as a benchmark performance of a suturing task. After watching the demonstration students' self-assessment scores displayed a very strong positive correlation with expert scores.

Feedback seeking

It is important that students learn how to seek feedback about their performance and how to take responsibility for seeking feedback from a range of sources. In the *Immediate Feedback* (IF) patient management programme (Harden et al., 1979) the learner was able to compare their management decisions with those of a subject matter expert and also with the decisions of a group of designated "good practitioners". Further feedback was also provided in relation to each response. Feedback provided from one source, in this case the subject expert, could be calibrated with the insights from another source, in this case the "good practitioner". Where feedback is obtained from multiple sources, self-assessment is likely to be more accurate.

It is important to note that the sources of feedback students draw on to facilitate the process of self-assessment are not limited to direct verbal/written feedback from teachers. Nicol (2021, p. 757) explores the importance of comparison for "internal feedback" defined as

The new knowledge that students generate when they compare their current knowledge and competence against some reference information.

Students draw on a wide range of sources in making the comparisons which form part of their internal feedback: teacher's comments, exemplars, rubrics, criteria, discussions in/outside class, blogs, videos, peer comments, and textbooks. Teachers can support students in this process by making suitable sources for comparison available to students.

Reflection

Students should evaluate the quality of their performance based on the feedback they have received, identifying their strengths and weaknesses; do they meet the required standards? Students should be given time to reflect on their achievements against the expected standards. After reflection students come to an evaluative judgement about their performance based on the criteria expected and the feedback they receive.

Self-reflection refers to a conscious mental process aimed at enhancing one's understanding of the problem as well judging the characteristics of his/her own performance. Such reflection process will lead to a self-assessment judgement which might be subject to further calibrations (Yan and Brown, 2017, p. 125).

Students are often encouraged to engage in reflection as an individual activity; however, it can also be useful to facilitate reflection through discussion with others (peers or a mentor). This may be something that students self-organise but can also be organised as part of the formal curriculum, for example, by timetabling and suggesting a focus for group reflection sessions.

Conclusion

Assessment is a key element of the education programme with students at the centre of the process. There is a need for a greater level of assessment literacy at all levels in a medical school with an understanding of the important role students can have as assessors. Students' involvement in assessment can enhance the effectiveness and quality of the education programme and at the same time can improve the quality of the student's learning. Students should have a voice in relation to both current and future assessment policy and implementation, with decisions taken through the lens of a student perspective.

Peer assessment and self-assessment are key roles for students as assessors. They can be seen from a pedagogical perspective, as a learning strategy promoting productive learning, as tools to assess abilities not readily measured by other assessment methods, and as the development of the person's skills to evaluate their own abilities.

The question is no longer whether students should be engaged with assessment, other than as the object of the assessment, but rather how students can best be involved in the assessment process.

References

Beaman, R., 1998. The unquiet…even loud, andragogy! Alternative assessments for adult learners. Innov. High. Educ. 23, 47–59.

Brown, G.T.L., Andrade, H.L., Chen, F., 2015. Accuracy in student self-assessment: Directions and cautions for research. Assess. Educ. 22 (4), 444–457.

Brown, G.T.L., Harris, L.R., 2013. Student self-assessment. In: McMillan, J.H. (Ed.), SAGE Handbook of Research on Classroom Assessment. SAGE, Los Angeles, California, USA. pp. 367–393.

Brown, G.T.L., Harris, L.R., 2014. The future of self-assessment in classroom practice: Reframing self-assessment as a core competency. Frontline Learn. Res. 3 (1), 22–30.

Cheng, W., Warren, M., 2000. Making a difference: Using peers to assess individual students' contributions to a group project. Teach. High. Educ. 5 (2), 243–255.

Costa, A.L., Kallick, B., 1992. In: Costa, A.L., Bellanca, J.A., Fogarty, R. (Eds.), If minds matter: A foreword to the future, Volume II.

Eva, K.W., Regehr, G., 2008. I'll never play professional football and other fallacies of self-assessment. J. Contin. Educ. Health. Prof. 28 (1), 14–19.

Falchikov, N., 2005. Improving Assessment Through Student Involvement. Routledge, London, UK.

Greenstein, L., Burke, M.A., 2020. Student-Engaged Assessment. Rowman and Littlefield, London, UK.

Harden, R.M., Dunn, W.R., Murray, T.S., Rogers, J., Stoane, C., 1979. Doctors accept a challenge: Self-assessment exercises in continuing medical education. BMJ. 2, 652.

Harden, R.M., Laidlaw, J.M., 1992. Effective continuing education: The CRISIS criteria. Med. Educ. 26 (5), 408–422.

Harden, R.M., Laidlaw, J.M., 2021. Essential Skills for a Medical Teacher (3rd ed). Elsevier, London, UK.

Harden, R.M., Lilley, P.M., 2018. The Eight Roles of the Medical Teacher. Elsevier, London, UK.

Hawkins, S.C., Osborne, A., Schofield, S.J., Pournaras, D.J., Chester, J.F., 2012. Improving the accuracy of self-assessment of practical clinical skills using video-feedback – the importance of including benchmarks. Med. Teach. 34 (4), 279–284.

Heron, J., 1981. Assessment revisited. In: Boud, D.J. (Ed.), Developing Student Autonomy in Learning. Kogan Page, London, UK.

Magin, D., 2001. Reciprocity as a source of bias in multiple peer-assessment of group work. Studies in higher education. Stud. High. Educ. 26 (1), 53–63.

McIntyre, K.R., Crawford, L.E., 2022. Outcomes for group working: Contextualising group work within professionalism frameworks. Med. Educ. 56 (5), 551.

Nicol, D., 2021. The power of internal feedback: Exploiting natural comparison processes. Assess. Eval. High. Edu. 46 (5), 756–778.

Norcini, J., Anderson, B., Bollela, V., et al., 2011. Criteria for good assessment: Consensus statement and recommendations from the Ottawa 2010 Conference. Med. Teach. 33 (3), 206–214.

Norcini, J., Anderson, M.B., Bollela, V., et al., 2018. 2018 Consensus framework for good assessment. Med. Teach. 40 (11), 1102–1109.

O'Donovan, B., Price, M., Rust, C., 2008. Developing student understanding of assessment standards: A nested hierarchy of approaches. Teach. High. Educ. 13 (2), 205–217.

PeerWise. University of Auckland, NZ. Accessed at: http://peerwise.cs.auckland.ac.nz/. Accessed 5th May 2022.

Portnoy, L., 2019. Designed to Learn. ASCD, USA.

Portnoy, L., 2019. Designed to Learn. Association for Supervision & Curriculum Development, Alexandria, Virginia, USA.

Quality Assurance Agency (QAA), 2018a. UK Quality Code for Higher Education, Part B: Assuring and Enhancing Academic Quality, Chapter B5: Student Engagement.

Quality Assurance Agency (QAA), 2018b. UK Quality Code for Higher Education, Part B: Assuring and Enhancing Academic Quality, Chapter B6: Assessment of Students and the Recognition of Prior Learning.

Rhind, S.M., MacKay, J., Brown, A.J., Mosley, C.J., Ryan, J.M., Hughes, K.J., Boyd, S., 2021. Developing Miller's Pyramid to support students' assessment literacy. J. Vet. Met. Educ. 48 (2), 158–162.

University of Reading, 2021. Engage in Assessment Online Toolkit: Peer Assessment. University of Reading, Reading, UK. https://www.reading.ac.uk/engageinas-sessment/peer-and-self-assessment/peer-assessment/eia-peer-assessment.aspx.

Wride, M., 2017. Guide to peer assessment. Academic Practice, University of Dublin Trinity College, ROI.

Yan, Z., 2018. Student self-assessment practices: The role of gender, school level, and goal orientation. Assess. Educ. 25 (2), 183–199.

Yan, Z., Brown, G.T.L., 2017. A cyclical self-assessment process: Towards a model of how students engage in self-assessment. Assess. Eval. High. Educ. 42 (8), 1247–1262.

Yan, Z., Brown, G.T.L., Lee, J.C.K., Qiu, X.L., 2020. Student self-assessment why do they do it. Educ. Psychol. 40 (4), 509–532.

Zimmerman, B.J., Schunk, D.H., 2011. Self-regulated learning and performance: An introduction and overview. In: Zimmerman, B.J., Schunk, D.H. (Eds.), A Handbook of Self-Regulation of Learning and Performance. Routledge, NYC, USA. pp. 1–14.

Zundert, M., Sluijsmans, D., Merriënboer, J., 2010. Effective peer assessment processes: Research findings and future directions. Learn. Instruct. 20 (4), 270–279.

9 | The student as a teacher

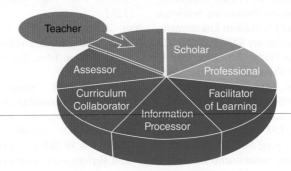

Student engagement as a teacher

Student engagement with the education programme, as described in this book, covers a range of activities, including curriculum development, assessment and facilitation of learning that relate to the role of the teacher. In this chapter, we focus directly on the role of the student as a teacher when the student serves as a peer teacher, a creator of learning resources, and a peer mentor (Figure 9.1).

The involvement of students as a teacher is now widely acknowledged as an important aspect of their educational experience (Dandavino et al., 2007). This may be part of the formal curriculum, and in some instances may even be an obligatory component. Student involvement in teaching can also be informal and extracurricular, such as tutorials organised by a student society or a student-led conference. In these cases, the instigation for the teaching may come from the students, from faculty, or as a partnership between students and faculty. There is also often a crossover between the roles related to teaching and the contexts in which these occur. What may begin as a student-led peer initiative, for example, informal peer teaching on LGBTQIA+ health, may then be incorporated by staff into the formal curriculum.

Peer teaching

Peer teaching sends a powerful message about the way students are perceived and their role in medical school.

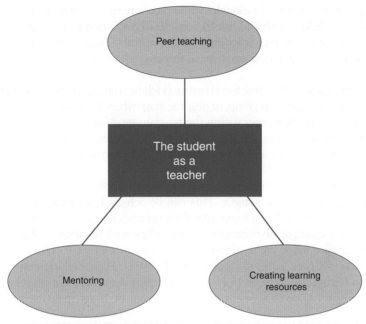

Figure 9.1 The roles of a student as a teacher.

> *It says to students 'you have knowledge worth sharing, you have a teacher's trust and you have an opportunity to support your friend's learning' (Lander, 2016).*

Peer teaching was defined by Topping (1996) as

> *People from similar social groupings who are not professional teachers helping each other to learn and learning themselves by teaching.*

While the role of the student as a teacher has gained momentum in recent years, the concept is not new. The value of students teaching students was accepted in the 19th Century. Laura Elizabeth Ingalls Wilder, best known as the author of a series of children's books including "Little House on the Prairie", was a teacher of young children while she was still a student at high school. On December 10, 1882, two months before her 16th birthday and still a student, she accepted a post for three terms as a teacher. With the increasing professionalisation of teaching, the teacher was recognised as someone usually older and with years of accumulated experience in the area being taught; consequently, the student as a teacher became less acceptable.

Peer teaching, however, is now common in medical schools as an adjunct to the established teaching programme. A survey in 2010 found that 76% of USA medical schools utilised some form of peer teaching in their medical programme (Soriano et al., 2010). There are different reasons for this growth (Burgess et al., 2014). Peer tutoring may reflect the interests of students to promote a particular topic but may also reflect a perceived gap in the curriculum. Indeed, research highlights that practical challenges including staff resources can be a factor that drives the adoption of peer tutoring. This is a somewhat controversial rationale; while there are many benefits of peer teaching that we discuss below, it should not be considered a solution to resource constraints. The implementation of peer teaching within medical schools is also motivated by a recognition of the need to develop medical students' skills as teachers.

In peer teaching, the student (the tutor) instructs fellow students at the same stage, where students are in the same year group, or near the stage where the student teacher is one or more years ahead of the learner within the programme. Newly qualified junior doctors may teach medical students, but the term near-peer teaching is usually reserved for the situation when the teacher and the student are in the same phase of their education.

The student as a tutor has the responsibility for helping other students to develop their understanding of a specific subject. This can be achieved, for example, through the tutor delivering a tutorial on a topic, providing tutorials that cover a new theme in the curriculum (for example sustainability), or providing students with feedback regarding their performance following their participation in a mock OSCE. This is sometimes called *directional peer learning* (Topping et al., 2017). Peer teaching may occur in a large group setting (for example, in a lecture) but more commonly occurs in small group settings. In Box 9.1, we present a student's reflections on being an anatomy peer tutor.

Box 9.1 Student case study: being a near-peer teacher

Reflections on the experience of teaching as an anatomy peer tutor, by Shreya Gupta, University of Edinburgh

I've been a near-peer teacher (NPT) for 4 years, primarily through my work with the Edinburgh Student Anatomy Society. I think teaching experiences are beneficial for both personal and professional growth. Teaching has helped me improve my communication and interpersonal skills – I'm constantly thinking about how I can make students feel more confident in interacting with me during tutorials. Teaching has also made me more adaptable and creative. Every group of students had unique dynamics, and with experience, I have become better at navigating these – maintaining a balance between "the keen and the quiet", generating energy when they are fatigued and modifying the delivery of teaching based on the tutees' knowledge.

One challenge I experienced initially was seeing that students were too focussed on trying to take notes to actively engage with teaching. We started providing handouts before and after tutorials (with solutions) and reminded students that these are openly accessible regardless of attendance. This meant we had a self-selected cohort of tutees who weren't just there for extra notes but rather were more likely to be "present" and engaging, with the comfort of knowing they would have access to resources after the session.

More recently, my role has extended into organising tutorials and mentoring NPTs. I encourage NPTs to move away from didactic teaching and reassure them that near-peer teaching is meant for the mutual benefit of learners and teachers; they are allowed to not know everything; they are allowed to make mistakes. From feedback, I've found that this reassurance goes a long way in making them perceive this teaching experience as an opportunity to explore themselves as educators, rather than a stressful 20-minute slot of rattling through dense slides.

Looking back, I can see how much I have grown as a learner and educator with every experience. Being an NPT and mentor is very much a part of my identity at medical school, and I find students emailing me for help even out with tutorials. Near-peer teaching is an invaluable tool, and I would highly encourage students to engage in both receiving and, importantly, delivering peer teaching.

The student teacher will tend to have a less expansive knowledge base than the faculty, is unlikely to be a subject expert, and will have less developed skills and less experience in teaching. Two or more tutors may lead peer tutorial sessions to provide additional peer support and to reduce the chance of idiosyncratic teaching (Ross and Cameron, 2007). The more competent and knowledgeable peer tutor manages and guides learning for the less competent, novice peer tutor (Topping et al., 2017). As noted by McLuckie and Topping (2004), however, peer teaching

> Should not be a diluted version of professional pedagogy but instead be specifically designed to capitalise on the different and complementary advantages of peer interaction.

Feedback from the tutor to the tutees is an important element of peer teaching.

> As the learning relationship develops, both helper and helped should begin to become more consciously aware of what is happening to them in their learning interaction and consequently, more able to monitor and regulate the effectiveness of their own learning strategies in different contexts (McLuckie and Topping, 2004, p. 569).

The peer tutor also acts as a role model –

> Modelling of enthusiasm and competence and the simple possibility of success by the helper could influence the self-confidence of the helped (McLuckie and Topping, 2004, p. 568).

As a role model, the peer teacher can convey what lies ahead – the hidden curriculum – and what is required to survive the programme. As described in Box 9.2, the peer teacher-student interaction can be formal, although even then a more informal atmosphere stimulates more interaction between students and the near-peer teacher. Near-peer teachers often work with students in a less formal, extracurricular

---

Box 9.2 An example of near-peer teaching at the University of Adelaide

From *Khaw, C., Raw, L., 2016. The outcomes and acceptability of near-peer teaching among medical students in clinical skills. Int. J. Med. Educ. 7, 188–194.*

In Year Six of the Adelaide MBBs curriculum, students are offered a formal medical education rotation; students tutor year 1-2 students in clinical skills for 16 hours per week (4 weeks). Activities include the teaching and facilitation of large and small groups, the teaching of history-taking and physical examination skills, the provision of feedback to junior peers, and the identification and remediation of underperforming peers. The student tutors provide formative feedback to peers, write and mark examination questions, and act as examiners for end-of-year OSCEs.

An evaluation of the programme demonstrated benefits for both the peer tutors and the students. For example, one student tutor said: "The elective not only provides me an opportunity to better my clinical skills, leadership skills and teamwork capabilities, but it also provides me with a rare and honoured glimpse into medical teaching and has made me more enthusiastic and interested in it."

setting, for example, helping students to prepare for an examination with a mock OSCE (see student case study examples in Chapters 6 and 8 – prescribing safety assessment; mock OSCEs).

Peer clinical teaching

Peer teaching was introduced initially in more theory-based classes in classroom settings. Its value is now also recognised in clinical teaching and learning. Peer teaching (Yu, 2011) can be effective to address:

- History taking
- Physical examination
- Practical procedures
- Procedural skills, for example, lumbar puncture
- Communication with patients

Peer teaching in the clinical context can enhance reflective learning both for the tutor and the tutee. Tutors feel more self-confident and acquire a deeper understanding of content (Nomura et al., 2017; Tai et al., 2014).

A simulated patient

Students may take on the role of a simulated patient and in this role provide feedback to students with regard to their performance in history taking or physical examination. In Chapter 8, we presented a student's reflections on taking on the role of a simulated patient.

Student-run clinics

The importance and relevance of student-run clinics have been recognised to simultaneously provide students with experience in teaching and in patient care. Senior students may find it helpful to work with a more junior student to encourage them to critically think about patient care (Hamso et al., 2012).

Recruitment and training peer teachers

Most peer teaching opportunities are offered to students on a voluntary basis, although how students are recruited is often not clearly described in published work (Burgess et al., 2014). It is possible to select applicants, for example, based on previous tutoring experience and accomplishments (Weyrich et al., 2008). The motivation to become involved in peer teaching is often the intrinsic rewards it can offer, and we describe such benefits below. It is not common for students to be financially rewarded for peer teaching (Burgess et al., 2014), although there are some examples of this (Nikendei et al., 2009; Weyrich et al., 2008). We have noted in earlier chapters that some students' involvement in particular roles may be limited by the lack of financial compensation for their time.

To support the role of peer teachers, many schools now offer training to students There is considerable variability in the duration of training from three-hour to two-year programmes, although most do include opportunities to practise teaching skills (Burgess et al., 2018).

The benefits of peer teaching

There is a growing body of research supporting the value of the student as a teacher and the benefits both to the student being taught and to the student who is teaching (Ross and Cameron, 2007).

Benefits to the student being taught (the tutee)

- Students can learn effectively. A systematic review of randomised studies of peer-assisted learning (PAL) concluded that "medical students experiencing PAL benefit in terms of academic performance, relative to those not receiving PAL" (Brierley et al., 2021).
- Students may learn better from another student who has a recent similar learning experience and understands their colleague's needs and how the content can be addressed to meet these needs (Box 9.3). As noted by Ignatio Estrado, "if a student can't learn the way we teach, maybe we should teach the way they learn".
- Students may feel more comfortable learning from a peer than from an expert teacher (ten Cate and Durning, 2007). The peer teacher may be less intimidating and create a less pressured learning environment in which students may be more prepared to ask questions or admit to gaps in their understanding (Nelson et al., 2013).

The benefits to the student teacher (the tutor)

- The student teacher gains academically and deepens their own learning (Duran and Topping, 2017). The student teacher may not have fully grasped a concept until they have had to explain it to others. As the Robert Heinlein quote goes, "When one teaches, two learn". In Box 9.4, we present reflections from a student's experience of teaching sex and relationship education within secondary schools.
- Teaching is an important role for the doctor and a key component of medical practice; the doctor is a teacher of patients and trainees. The word doctor is derived from the Latin doceo, "I teach". Teaching has been affirmed as a necessary skill for students by accredited bodies, for example, the General Medical Council in the UK and the Liaison Committee on Medical Education in the USA. Peer teaching can help to prepare a student for their teaching responsibilities as a physician, "it was only after they taught medicine related material that students saw the benefit of teaching as a way of preparing for becoming a physician and not merely as a way to review or help their peers" (Amorosa et al., 2011).

Box 9.3   The benefits of peer teaching

The student as a teacher may result in more effective learning than traditional approaches

My (RMH) granddaughter, who lives in Spain, was approached by the mother of a pupil in the same class. He had consistently failed the maths examination and because of this was not allowed to progress. In desperation, Alba was asked if she would coach the boy. She agreed to help, and in sessions with the boy, she discovered that there were some basic essential principles (I suppose we would call these threshold concepts) he had not grasped, which he had not felt he could express to the teachers. Alba, having studied the subject herself, explained these to him in a way that he understood. To everyone's surprise and delight, he passed the next maths exam comfortably and was able to proceed.

Box 9.4 Student case study: learning through teaching sex and relationships education in secondary schools

An example of a teaching experience with the university, by Margherita Vianello, University of Edinburgh

One of the university experiences I enjoyed the most was teaching sex and relationships education (SRE) in secondary schools through the charity Sexpression. I worked as a Lesson Planner, so I wrote the material that I and other volunteers delivered. SRE is not compulsory in Scottish schools, and therefore there is no specific guidance on what should be covered, including no resources on which to base lessons. We generally had a lot of freedom in deciding how to tackle the topics schools requested we teach. This taught me to be flexible with where I look for information; there would never be one single book or website that contained all the information I was looking for. As sex and relationships grew to be a huge area of interest for me, it also led me to build up a bank of resources that I accumulated organically in everyday life, mostly through talks at Sexpression and my all-consuming love of podcasts.

This impacted the way I see myself learning in medicine too; medicine can feel really overwhelming, as any given topic is vast, and it can be difficult to know what level of knowledge is necessary for exams. However, I think teaching with Sexpression showed me that you also gain knowledge more organically, particularly in the areas you have a specific interest. I have certainly noticed this reflected in learning medicine, as I seem to always learn so much more from placements in specialities I have an attraction towards, despite the exact same number of hours being spent in the hospital as those specialities that I do not feel quite so positively about. It makes me feel quite excited at the prospect of specializing in something I really love.

- A further benefit is that students who engage in teaching gain insights and an understanding of a teacher's job, which helps to develop empathy between the student and teacher. When reflecting on their peer tutoring, one student reported to the authors that it "let me see what works go into teaching; and it's a lot!"
- Peer teaching can be satisfying for the student teacher and result in greater self-esteem and self-confidence. For some student teachers, there is an intrinsic enjoyment in teaching, and in developing the skills associated with that role. The fact that the student has a role to play in the delivery of the programme may also result in positive feelings.

Benefits to the education programme
- Peer teaching, as part of the curriculum delivery, supports the idea of a collaborative learning environment in the school, encouraging teamwork and collaboration as an expected learning outcome (Topping et al., 2017).
- While of benefit to all students, peer teaching may also help a school to respond to the requirements of a more diverse group of students with the need for more learning support. In Box 9.5, we present an example of a student-led society that offers peer tutoring to students from non-traditional backgrounds before entry and in the early years of medical school.
- Student-led peer teaching can provide additional learning opportunities that it may not be possible to provide within the formal curriculum. Schools should be careful, however, about relying on peer teaching to fill gaps arising due to resource limitations. While this may be of immediate benefit to the programme, it may not in the longer term be a solution to the issues faced.

Box 9.5 Student case study: accessibility in medicine society

A student reflects on the development of a peer mentor and tutoring scheme to support students from non-traditional backgrounds, by Alex Clark, University of Edinburgh

Patients deserve diverse doctors – this was the ethos behind Accessibility in Medicine (AIM). AIM was conceived as a student-led society addressing socioeconomic inequality in medical education at a local level. It targeted areas of disparity that were difficult to address on a grander scale by existing widening participation schemes. This included facilitating one-to-one mentorship for local high school pupils applying to medical school. Recognising that those who have faced barriers prior to university would not see those obstacles miraculously resolved upon acceptance, we also worked to maintain a continuity of support once their studies began. To this end, we provided free, peer-led tutorials to pre-clinical students. My role in AIM, as its founder and president, was overseeing a committee of volunteers without whom the project would never have succeeded. With their direction, AIM flourished.

There were a number of challenges throughout AIM's conception and development, not least of which was the mammoth task of developing and delivering a curriculum of educational resources and tutorials. However, the hurdle I least expected was the last one I faced. As I grew closer to graduation, the question of long-term sustainability arose. While it was clear that the society needed new ideas and perspectives to be viable, stepping away from AIM was personally and emotionally difficult. The society had been my passion project for years and giving up control of it was no easy task.

I struggled with the need to move on from AIM, but I have never regretted doing so – it continues to move forward without me and is stronger for it. Today, we know of at least one volunteer involved that was a high school mentee years prior. My experiences as a teacher in AIM were immensely fulfilling, and I look back on them with pride.

Creation of learning resources

A less frequent focus for peer teaching has been the student as a creator, or often co-creator, of learning resources (see Chapter 7 for a more general discussion of the student as co-creator). This teaching role has assumed added importance with increasing interest in, and adoption of educational approaches that require the provision of online learning resources. For example, in a flipped learning approach the student will engage in some learning activities, often offered as online resources, prior to coming to class. The COVID-19 pandemic has necessitated the greater use of online learning, and there are opportunities for students to become involved in the development of learning resources. Indeed, Prensky (2001) who introduced the terms "digital native" and "digital immigrant" argued for greater involvement of students, particularly in the creation of learning resources.

> *The single biggest problem facing education today is that our digital immigrant instructors who speak an outdated language (that of the predigital age) are struggling to teach a population that speaks an entirely new language.*

The resources produced by students can include:

- An online mini-lecture on a topic
- A set of notes on a subject with further reading material
- A set of PowerPoint slides with an attached commentary

Box 9.6   The Dental Wikipedia Editing Project

The Dental Wikipedia Editing Project, with support from the Cochrane Collaboration, is an online editable encyclopaedia that was launched in 2017 at the Dundee Dental School. It now involves dental schools worldwide, including several schools in the UK, North America, Canada, and Asia. The School of Dentistry at the International Medical University (IMU), Malaysia became a member of the project in 2019 when students were trained by accredited peer editors from Dundee to appraise and edit the literature on subjects relevant to dental education. Students also developed a host of learning skills, including information literacy and critical thinking in an active and collaborative pedagogical approach. Following training, topics of interest were generated, reviewed, and approved by a student-led committee for scripting and publication on the Dental Wikipedia website. Shortlisted articles were presented at the annual Dental Wikipedia Conference. Students from IMU were awarded The WCODS Cochrane Oral Health Innovation Poster Award at the 2020 Conference.

Source: https://blog.dundee.ac.uk/one-dundee/dundee-dental-wiki-edit/.

- An interactive computer programme
- A virtual patient or patient-management problem
- Interactive quizzes

The benefits of student co-creation of learning resources

The production of learning resources is a valuable learning activity and goes back to Dewey's idea (1938) of learning by doing. The benefits of students' involvement in co-creating learning resources include (Egbert, 2017, Chapter 7):

- A gain in subject knowledge
- Communication skills
- Critical thinking, reasoning, and creativity
- Collaboration skills

Students can create learning resources in areas where they or faculty have identified a learning need. An example was the need for resources relating to the topic of climate change and sustainability as reported by students, which led to students at the University of Cambridge "working to produce an educational manual for students and junior doctors on sustainable healthcare and the health implications of climate change" (Green and Legard, 2020).

The creation of learning resources can be a team activity with students working in collaboration with peers and/or with faculty, in the various stages of the development process. An example of a student/staff collaboration on the creation of a Dental Wikipedia website is given in Box 9.6. Where there are classes associated with the learning resources, students can also be involved in peer teaching. In the example of sustainable healthcare given above, Green and Legard argued that "student teachers should be central to the organization and delivery of both lectures and small group teaching".

Peer mentoring

Mentorship is one of the core roles of a medical teacher (Harden and Lilley, 2018). Peer mentorship differs from peer teaching because it does not involve a deliberate didactic element (Altonji et al., 2019). Peer mentoring is a relationship between students where one student, the peer mentor, who has successfully negotiated a particular stage in their studies, supports one or more students, the mentee. The mentor is a trusted counsel and guide and provides support and advice over a period of time. Although not exclusively, peer mentoring is often adopted to support students' transition during the first year at university.

The role of the student mentor

The role of a student mentor may vary from institution to institution and may include (Adolphus, 2010):

- Orientation, familiarisation, and giving advice about the university and aspects of university life.
- Acting as facilitator and advisor of the skills needed to survive university life, for example, time management and study skills.
- Identifying when a student is experiencing difficulties and developing with them a plan to overcome the difficulties including, when necessary, referral to support services available on medical health or financial matters.
- Providing moral support and friendship, encouraging the mentee and helping boost their self-esteem.

Mentorship skills

The skills and qualities needed to be an effective student mentor include (Adolphus, 2010):

- A commitment to the relationship
- Active listening skills
- Providing the mentee with undivided attention
- Not being judgemental
- Assisting the mentee to work through problems and produce appropriate solutions
- Empathy and putting yourself in another person's shoes and feeling what they are feeling
- Remembering that you are not the mentee's only source of support
- Confidentiality

The benefits of mentorship

Students can benefit from being mentors and mentees (Ramani et al., 2006). In Boxes 9.7 and 9.8, we present two students' reflections on their roles as mentors. In a review of the literature on peer mentoring in medical school, benefits for mentees were identified as including stress reduction and ease of transition: both mentees and mentors benefitted from professional and personal development (Akinla et al., 2018). The 'peer' aspect of mentoring has also been highlighted as significant in creating an informal and relatable context within which students feel comfortable discussing emotions and seeking support (de Vries-Erich et al., 2016; Altonji et al., 2019).

Box 9.7 Student case study: mentoring through the lived experience of illness

A student reflects on sharing their experiences of mental illness, by Usama Ali, University College London

During Medical School, I was admitted as a patient in a psychiatric facility. The experience taught me the realities of being a medical student with severe mental illness. In particular, the hard lessons of how stigmatised mental illnesses are amongst medical students became apparent.

As a result of these experiences, I started sharing my experiences with other medical students and doctors. The aim of this was to make other medical students who were in a similar position to me feel less alone, although I also hope to make students feel a bit more prepared for their psychiatry placements.

To raise awareness, I run a blog and have given various talks. Venues for these talks have included various Medical School Psychiatry Societies, the BMA, and the British Islamic Medical Association. More recently, I have worked with the Psychiatric Trainees Committee (part of the Royal College of Psychiatrists) to discuss how best to support doctors/medical students with mental illness.

This has been a unique teaching experience. Often, displaying signs of vulnerability as a teacher is discouraged. This project, however, has required me to completely embrace my own vulnerability whilst sharing it with others. Although I have found it difficult and emotionally challenging at times, it is also incredibly rewarding. Receiving "thank-you" messages from medical students who feel more empowered to seek help following my talks is heart-warming.

Interestingly, after people hear my story, they often share their story of mental illness with me as well. On a personal level, this makes me feel less alone as well. We often forget that students can inspire the teacher as well, and it is humbling to be reminded of this.

Box 9.8 Student case study: mentoring on the medical peacework course

An example of peer mentoring on a course, by Victor Chelashow, Moi University School of Medicine (former chair and project coordinator for MSSR) http://www.medicalpeacework. org/mpw-courses.html

Medical Students for Social Responsibility (MSSR) is an organization of health sciences students at Moi University that aims to promote peace and health in communities through advocacy, outreach, and projects. MSSR organizes a Medical Peacework Course to promote an understanding of peace and violence and to lay a foundation for humanitarian, human rights, and medical peace work. Senior medical students who have already completed the course guide groups of students through near-peer mentorships. Groups are self-selected, so students choose colleagues with whom they feel most comfortable engaging. Mentors draw from their own experiences, prepare learning resources and are keen to facilitate but not instruct mentees. Mentees give feedback at the end of the courses on their experiences and areas for improvement.

The benefits of such interactions, including social and emotional support, create a safe space for open (and intriguing) discussions and engage participants in collaborative problem solving. The mentors hone their interpersonal and communication skills, consolidate their understanding of concepts on medical peace work and gain new perspectives. Furthermore, mentors have self-satisfaction from watching their mentees succeed in the courses and take on mentor roles.

By assuming the role of mentors and teachers and becoming more autonomous in their learning, medical students have made the MPW course (which is not part of the school curriculum) remain relevant and impact not just themselves but also the communities in which they act.

Box 9.9 Student case study: BAME medics peer mentoring scheme

An example of a mentoring scheme for students from Black, Asian, and Minority Ethnic backgrounds, by Vishwani Chauhan, University of Edinburgh

One of the greatest challenges during the COVID-19 pandemic was cultivating and sustaining a sense of social belonging in the face of isolation. This particularly affected people in the early stages of university. There are studies showing that BAME university students may make this group even more vulnerable to isolation at this time.

The BAME Medics Edinburgh mentor scheme was launched in September 2020 as a way to encourage academic and social connections between preclinical BAME medical students during the pandemic. We asked clinical medical students from BAME backgrounds to sign up to be mentors. They were required to submit brief informal bios as part of this process. We published around thirty such profiles on a form where potential mentees could rank their preferences. The form was sent out to preclinical medical students via social networking platforms and university website platforms. Based on everyone's preferences, we matched preclinical medical students with mentors from clinical years.

The scheme encouraged mentors and mentees to communicate regularly, and we hosted online movie nights and chats to encourage a social scene. This allowed pre-clinical students to also get to know one another. Mentors and mentees also formed lasting connections, allowing for advice and experiences to be exchanged. Feedback on the mentor scheme was collected halfway through the year and then at the end of the year and was very positive. The scheme is now being run for its second year and continues to be a source of belonging and community for BAME medical students in the early stages of university. With easing restrictions, social events have transitioned from online to face-to-face. We are delighted to have founded something that benefited students at a difficult time and continues to sustain itself in the form of lasting social bonds.

Peer mentoring can be particularly beneficial for groups who may feel a lack of belonging at university. In Box 9.9, a student reports on a peer mentoring scheme developed by the BAME Medics student group at the University of Edinburgh.

Implementation of peer teaching

The implementation of peer teaching requires careful planning and consideration by students and teachers. Ross and Cameron (2007) identify questions (Box 9.10) that should be addressed when implementing peer teaching. While the questions refer to "teaching", they are also applicable to mentoring. The issues to be addressed can be summarised as:

- What is the aim of peer teaching?
- Who are the tutors, and how are they trained?
- How are the tutor and tutees prepared for the learning interaction?
- What format will the interaction take?
- How will peer teaching be evaluated?
- How does peer teaching relate to the curriculum?
- How will the implementation of peer teaching be managed within the school?

Addressing these questions is helpful for students and faculty who wish to develop peer teaching or mentoring and who have little or no experience in the area but can also be useful to those with established peer teaching schemes, as a prompt to

Box 9.10 Key questions: implementing peer teaching

From *Ross, M.T., Cameron, H.S., 2007. Peer assisted learning: a planning and implementation framework: AMEE Guide No. 30. Med. Teach. 29 (6), 529.*

1. What is the current situation and context in the curriculum?
2. Why is this PAL project being considered now?
3. Who is responsible for the project and who will lead it?
4. What are the aims and objectives of the project for tutors?
5. What are the aims and objectives of the project for tutees?
6. What are the aims and objectives of the project for the institution?
7. Who will be tutors and how will they be recruited?
8. What training will tutors require and how will this be provided?
9. How else will tutors prepare themselves and reflect afterwards?
10. Who will be the tutees and how will they be recruited?
11. What related prior knowledge and experience will tutees have already?
12. What information and preparation will tutees require before the interaction?
13. What will be the format of the interaction, and what resources are required?
14. What would be a typical plan of activities during the PAL interaction?
15. When and where will PAL interactions occur, and how will they be arranged?
16. What feedback will be collected from participants and how will it be used?
17. How else will the project be piloted and evaluated?
18. What are the academic hypotheses and how will they be tested?
19. Who are the potential stakeholders in the project?
20. What are the staff time and funding implications of the project?
21. How could the project be developed, and how might it affect the curriculum?
22. What are the potential pitfalls or barriers to the success of this project?
23. What are the key points on the timeline for this project?
24. What actions need to be taken to develop the project, and by whom?

reflect on and potentially revise the scheme. Ongoing consideration should be given to the questions to ensure that peer teaching or mentoring is being used appropriately and remains of benefit to students.

Some aspects relating to the implementation of peer teaching and mentoring, raised by these questions, merit particular attention:

- *Agreement and clarity on aims:* The aim of peer teaching or mentoring, the responsibilities, and the expectations of those involved should be explicitly discussed, agreed upon, and described. This will ensure that the purpose of the peer teaching/mentoring, and where it fits within the curriculum or wider school provision, has been carefully considered. This can highlight opportunities for linking between teaching sessions (formal and informal) but can also flag up concerns, for example, where extracurricular peer teaching or mentorship is being used to address gaps in the curriculum or student support provided by the school. It may be useful to revisit this agreement periodically to ensure that it still applies, particularly where there are concerns about how peer teaching or mentoring is working in practice.
- *Develop a peer teaching culture:* There is a need to establish a culture where peer teaching is welcomed; that teaching is a powerful learning experience and should be recognised and promoted. Even where this is recognised, the

culture of the medical school may be teacher-centred and not supportive of peer teaching. In addition, students may question the role of students as teachers and whether this practice is of educational or financial value. Colvin noted that "peer tutors have to convince the other students in the classes that though they were students just like everyone else they had additional insight and credibility that allowed them to function as a resource apart from the instructional staff" (Colvin 2007, p. 174). However, the "convincing" should not rest with the peer tutors; rather it is the responsibility of the school to ensure that peer teaching is embedded in the curriculum and that the value of peer teaching is explained to students and faculty.

- *Minimise barriers to participation as teachers:* Students may find it challenging to teach or mentor while developing as doctors themselves (Hamso et al., 2012). Allocating time to be involved in the role of teacher may be more challenging for students who have caring responsibilities or are required to work alongside studying. It is important to remind student societies of this issue and encourage them to review the timing of teaching sessions to ensure they are widely accessible to all those who might want to be involved as tutors. Those organising peer teaching may also consider alternative forms of teaching engagement that are more flexible in their timing and required input, including the co-creation of learning resources. Where possible, it would be helpful for the school to secure funding to support peer teaching in order to minimise any financial barriers to participation as tutors.
- *Training tutors and mentors:* Emphasis should be placed on training the student teacher/mentor and providing ongoing support. Training should include sessions on the theory and practice of medical education. Students should also be supported to ensure that they are aware of and able to implement equality, diversity, and inclusion principles. As Burgess et al. (2018) note, "Knowledge and skills acquired during initial training programs require ongoing reinforcement and practice, which may be best achieved by embedding and marrying more peer teacher training and PAL opportunities within curricula".
- *Developing reflective teachers:* Students should be supported to become reflective teachers. After each peer teaching session, encourage students to allow time for reflection and consideration of what, if any, changes need to be made before the next session. Discussion of the experience with other tutors or with faculty may also be helpful in promoting reflection. It may also be useful to consider developing a more formal Peer Observation of Teaching (POT) programme (Rees et al., 2015). Reflections on a student-led pilot of a POT programme at the University of Edinburgh are given in Chapter 8.

Conclusions

The student's involvement as a teacher is an important role through which they contribute directly to the teaching programme. While many wider aspects of a teacher's role are addressed in other chapters, here we have considered students as peer teachers, as creators of learning resources, and as peer mentors.

Peer teaching has been widely documented and has been shown to have benefits for both the peer teacher (the tutor) and the student tutees. Connected to their role as curriculum collaborator, students can also contribute to teaching through the development of learning resources. Engaging in more of a support for a teaching role, the student can also act as a peer mentor for one or more students with evidence of the benefit for mentor and mentee.

While peer teaching can bring many benefits to the students involved and to the school, careful consideration should be given to potential challenges when implementing a peer teaching programme, including clarity on the aims, fit within the school, and training of all those involved.

References

Adolphus, M., 2010. How To Be a Peer Mentor. Emerald Publishing, Bingley, UK.

Akinla, O., Hagan, P., Atiomo, W., 2018. A systematic review of the literature describing the outcomes of near-peer mentoring programs for first year medical students. BMC Med. Educ. 18, 98.

Altonji, S.J., Baños, J.H., Harada, C.N., 2019. Perceived benefits of a peer mentoring program for first-year medical students. Teach. Learn. Med. 31 (4), 445–452.

Amorosa, J.M.H., Mellman, L.A., Graham, M.J., 2011. Medical students as teachers: How preclinical teaching opportunities can create an early awareness of the role of physician as teacher. Med. Teach. 33 (2), 137–144.

Brierley, C., Ellis, L., Reid, E.R., 2021. Peer-assisted learning in medical education: A systematic review and meta-analysis. Med. Educ. 56 (4), 365–373.

Burgess, A., McGregor, D., 2018. Peer teacher training for health professional students: A systematic review of formal programs. BMC Med. Educ. 18, 263.

Burgess, A., McGregor, D., Mellis, C., 2014. Medical students as peer tutors: A systematic review. BMC Med. Educ. 14, 115.

Colvin, J.W., 2007. Peer tutoring and social dynamics in higher education. Mentor Tutor. 15 (2), 165–181.

Dandavino, M., Snell, L., Wiseman, J., 2007. Why medical students should learn how to teach. Med. Teach. 29 (6), 558–565.

de Vries-Erich, J.M., Dornan, T., Boerboom, T.B., Jaarsma, A.D., Helmich, E., 2016. Dealing with emotions: Medical undergraduates' preferences in sharing their experiences. Med. Educ. 50 (8), 817–828.

Dewey, J., 1938. Experience and Education. Macmillan Company, New York, USA.

Duran, D., Topping, K., 2017. Learning by Teaching: Evidence-Based Strategies to Enhance Learning in the Classroom. Routledge, London, UK.

Egbert, J., 2017. Chapter 7: Supporting student production. In: Egbert, J. (Ed.). Methods of Education Technology: Principles, Practice, and Tools. Pressbooks, Montreal, Canada.

Green, M., Legard, C., 2020. Peer-teaching could help bring sustainable healthcare into the medical education curriculum. Med. Teach. 42 (5), 598–599.

Hamso, M., Ramsdell, A., Balmer, D., Boquin, C., 2012. Medical students as teachers at CoSMO, Columbia University's student-run clinic: A pilot study and literature review. Med. Teach. 34 (3), e189–e197.

Harden, R., Lilley, P., 2018. The Eight Roles of the Medical Teacher. Elsevier, London, UK.

Khaw, C., Raw, L., 2016. The outcomes and acceptability of near-peer teaching among medical students in clinical skills. Int. J. Med. Educ. 7, 188–194.

Lander, J., 2016. Students as Teachers. Harvard: Usable Knowledge. https://www.gse.harvard.edu/uk/blog/students-teachers.

McLuckie, J., Topping, K.J., 2004. Transferable skills for online peer learning. Assess. Eval. High. Educ. 29 (5), 563–584.

Nelson, A.J., Nelson., S.V., Linn, A.M.J., Raw, L.E., Kildea, H.B., Tonkin, A.L., 2013. Tomorrow's educators…today? Implementing near-peer teaching for medical students. Med. Teach. 35 (2), 156–159.

Nikendei, C., Andreesen, S., Hoffmann, K., Jünger, J., 2009. Cross-year peer tutoring on internal medicine wards: Effects on self-assessed clinical competencies–A group control design study. Med. Teach. 31 (2), e32–e35.

Nomura, O., Onishi, H., Kato, H., 2017. Medical students can teach communication skills - a mixed methods study of cross-year peer tutoring. BMC Med. Educ. 17 (1), 103. Erratum in: BMC Med. Educ. 17(1), 187.

Prensky, M., 2001. Digital natives. Digital immigrants part 1. On the Horizon. 9 (5), 1–6.

Ramani, S., Gruppen, L., Kachur, E.K., 2006. Twelve tips for developing effective mentors. Med. Teach. 28 (5), 404–408.

Rees, E.L., Davies, B., Eastwood, M., 2015. Developing students' teaching through peer observation and feedback. Perspect. Med. Educ. 4, 268–271.

Ross, M.T., Cameron, H.S., 2007. Peer assisted learning: A planning and implementation framework: AMEE Guide No. 30. Med. Teach. 29 (6), 527–545.

Soriano, R.P., Blatt, B., Coplit, L., 2010. Teaching medical students how to teach: A national survey of students-as-teachers programs in U.S. medical schools. Acad. Med. 85 (11), 1725–1731.

Tai, J.H.M., Haines, T.P., Canny, B.J., Molloy, E.K., 2014. A study of medical students' peer learning on clinical placements: What have they taught themselves to do. J. Peer Learn. 7, 57–80.

ten Cate, O., Durning, S., 2007. Dimensions and psychology of peer teaching in medical education. Med. Teach. 29 (6), 546–552.

Topping, K., Buchs, C., Duran, D., van Keer, H., 2017. Effective peer learning: From principles to practical implementation. Taylor and Francis, London, UK.

Topping, K.J., 1996. The effectiveness of peer tutoring in further and higher education: A typology and review of the literature. High. Educ. 32, 321–345.

Weyrich, P., Schrauth, M., Kraus, B., Habermehl, D., Netzhammer, N., Zipfel, S., Jünger, J., Riessen, R., Nikendei, C., 2008. Undergraduate technical skills training by student tutors: Tutees' acceptance and tutors' attitudes. BMC Med. Educ. 8, 18.

Yu, T.-C., Wilson, N.C., Singh, P.P., Lemanu, D.P., Hawken, S.J., Hill, A.G., 2011. Medical students-as-teachers: A systematic review of peer-assisted teaching during medical school. Adv. Med. Educ. Pract. 2, 157–172.

10 | The student as a scholar

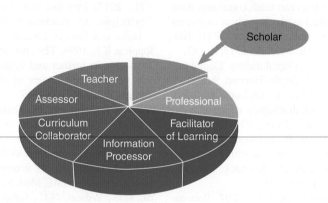

Every student is a scholar

"Dear Educators: Every student is a scholar" was the headline of an article by Daniel Jean (2018), the Executive Director of the Educational Opportunity Fund Program and Academic Development at Montclair State University in New Jersey. He argued that all learners should be seen as "scholars" rather than as students as this boosts the learner's perceptions of their academic perspectives and promotes a culture where they are expected to flourish academically.

The old English word *"scholere"*, meaning *"student"*, derives from the medieval and late-Latin word *"scholaris"*, meaning *"of or belonging to a school"*. The terms student and scholar have long been used interchangeably. Yet there are potential differences in the application of these labels that raise some interesting questions in relation to student roles.

In the USA, one school district has addressed this explicitly. Their students (elementary, middle school, and high school) are referred to as *"scholars,"* and they draw an explicit distinction between student and scholar: students, it is suggested, are teacher-driven, dependent, uncertain learners, learning passively from the teacher, while scholars are peer-driven, engaged, multifaceted learners, collaborators, problem-solvers who are self-motivated, passionate, independent, and innovative (www.fwps.org/domain/1712).

By placing an emphasis on the educational aspect of their work and learning, scholars is not only appropriate, it is a way for the school district to emphasise the value and importance the students have and the work they put in (Federal Way Public Schools 2017).

Palmer provided a deeper understanding of learning practices and how students achieve *"scholar status"*.

Implicit in these definitions however are notions of dependence and independence. Students are often considered to be dependent on their teachers or advisors while scholars are viewed as functioning and learning independently of such agents (Palmer 2016, p. 219).

While we do not agree with such a clear dichotomy, indeed we have presented many examples in the chapters of this book that demonstrate that students are not passive or dependent, it is useful to reflect on the ways in which students can also be scholars and what this student role involves. Though not referring specifically to students, Cleland defined scholarship in education as

Publicly disseminated activities that advance practice and knowledge for health professions educators and/or the health professions education community (Cleland et al., 2021).

We have explored in earlier chapters in this book the role of a student as an information seeker, a facilitator of their own learning, a curriculum developer, an assessor, and as a teacher. There are benefits to be gained if these roles are approached from the perspective of a scholar.

Participation as a student scholar can:

- Offer students a wider perspective on their learning, going beyond that which is required to succeed in the programme
- Position the students as significant agents of change
- Lead to recognition of the student's performance as a scholar, for example, through publication of work, and this can contribute to career progression
- Extend students' engagement as a member of the wider community of health professionals with an interest in medical education
- Open new opportunities, such as eligibility for grants to support their work, for example, through an AMEE student innovation award

Every student can be a scholar. However, what aspects of scholarship students are interested in and how this is applied will vary. It should also be noted that where the requirements of scholarship are not part of the formal education programme, the challenges for student engagement and participation that we have noted in earlier chapters will also apply, and for some students extra-curricular, unpaid work is not possible due to other work or caring responsibilities.

The scholarship of teaching

In *The Eight Roles of the Medical Teacher* (Harden and Lilley, 2018), we argue that teachers are not simply technicians responsible for applying prescribed approaches to curriculum planning, teaching and assessment. There is, as described by Boyer (1990), a Scholarship of Teaching. Boyer argues that there has been too narrow a definition of scholarship around research-based activities and advocates the need for a broader definition of scholarship that included teaching. Teachers can demonstrate scholarship by reflecting on their teaching, innovating and bringing about change where necessary, applying an evidence-informed approach to their teaching practice, and communicating their experiences to other teachers.

Given the increasing involvement of students as peer teachers (Chapter 9), scholarship of teaching should not just be the prerogative of the teacher but should also be seen as a role for the student. Indeed, scholarship in education can be seen as a manifestation of the growing interest and engagement of students in medical education. For example, as we described in Chapter 1, there has been a significant increase in the number of students contributing as an author or co-author to publications in the journal *Medical Teacher*.

We noted in the last chapter that there is a broad range in the training offered to students to support them as peer teachers. While some training focuses on providing students with opportunities to practise teaching skills, others encourage students to engage with educational theory and evidence as underpinning their teaching practice. Not all students may wish to become scholars in medical education; however, it is important to support those whose interests lie in this area. The University of Edinburgh offers a two-year mentorship and training programme – the Undergraduate Certificate of Medical Education – in which students are mentored by an experienced educator, work collaboratively in small peer groups, and attend a series of medical education workshops. In Box 10.1, we present a reflection from one of the students on this programme.

There is also a growing number of organisations that support and provide a community of practice for student medical educators including the Junior Association for the Study of Medical Education; the Developing Medical Educators Group; the Medical Student Alliance for Global Education; and the International Federation of Medical Students Association. Schools can support students by publicising these and other opportunities for students to connect with and receive support as they develop as medical educational scholars. There may also be opportunities for students to apply for formal recognition of their expertise in teaching and learning. For example, student members of AMEE (Association for Medical Education in Europe) can apply for recognition as Associate Fellows. In the UK, students can apply to Advance HE for Associate Fellow of the Higher Education Academy. While fees related to such memberships and applications are often reduced for students, it may still be a barrier for some. Schools may consider a fund to support student membership.

Box 10.1 Student case study: developing scholarship in teaching

A student reflects on his experience studying for the Undergraduate Certificate in Medical Education, by Wesley McLoughlin, University of Edinburgh

Education lies at the heart of any career in medicine, starting, but certainly not ending, in medical school. I was fortunate, during my undergraduate years, to have the opportunity to join the Undergraduate Certificate in Medical Education (UGCME) programme. This related to aspects of medical education that we were already involved in but also gave me early exposure to different concepts and pedagogical models.

The programme educated us in foundational concepts, enabling us to become more intentional with what and how we teach. It gave us opportunities to hear from eminent educators and take part in research locally. Thanks to the reflective components and 1:1 tutor mentorship, it also created a helpful feedback dynamic which allowed adapting techniques and strategies. This continuous modulation and improvement cycle has given me a growing passion, in particular for asking for teaching feedback.

More often than not (and I have certainly been guilty of this) feedback is a final thought, using a boilerplate structure. But learning to ask some simple questions has paid dividends in terms of the resulting useful feedback. For example, (i) What do I want to find out? (ii) What will responses to this question help with? (iii) Will asking this question in a particular way potentially limit responses?

Then the answers are, of course, constrained by the short attention span of responding students (like myself!). The UGCME has given me a head start into what I hope will be a lifelong passion and interest in educating and being educated.

Demonstration of scholarship

While working on their study programme and mastering the course content to achieve the expected learning outcomes, the student can demonstrate scholarship in a number of ways (Figure 10.1).

- *Reflecting* on their experience in the education programme, considering what works, what doesn't work, and explanations for each item
- *Reviewing* the school's approach to curriculum planning, teaching and learning, and assessment from an evidence-based perspective. Does the evidence available suggest that the best approaches have been adopted?
- *Supporting innovation* and the introduction of new approaches to the different elements of the education programme
- *Undertaking research* in relation to aspects of the education programme with a view to illuminating the value of the different features
- *Communicating* their experience and the lessons learned to the different stakeholders
- *Engagement in a research project* on a foundation science or clinical theme as an elective, required part of the course or extra-curricular activity

The reflective student

The student can reflect on their experience as a learner in lectures, small group discussions, and clinical teaching, and on their experience with the assessment programme and the feedback provided. This experience may offer new insights into the

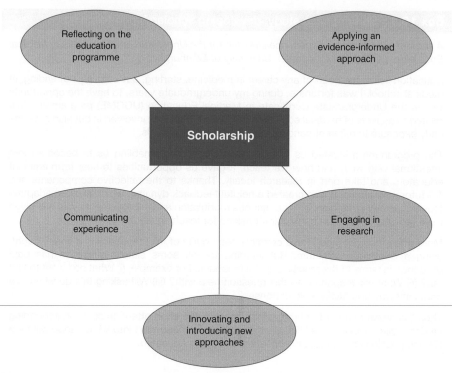

Figure 10.1 Demonstration of scholarship.

curriculum and learning programme. With some understanding of and scholarly engagement with education principles, students can interpret their experiences and ideas through the lens of theory. For example, could learning be made more effective if the FAIR principles were applied with the provision of meaningful feedback, active rather than passive learning, individualisation of learning, and an emphasis on relevance (Harden and Laidlaw, 2012)? Are the assessment approaches matched to the expected learning outcomes and the learning methods, and do they provide a reliable and valid assessment of the students' competence?

The student should be encouraged to disengage at times temporarily from the immediacy of learning a topic and to reflect on the education programme. Students are frequently asked to review the education programme and to provide their perspective on the teaching, learning, and assessment through course evaluation questionnaires or focus group discussions (as discussed in Chapter 7). Scholarly reflections go beyond the standard feedback responses and involve students relating their experience to broader discussions within medical education. End-of-course evaluations may not be the best format in which to gather such reflections. Instead, there may be an open call for comments, a dialogue facilitated on a specific issue in a course about which there is a concern. Students who are interested can be invited to prepare a paper or a review of the topic, in which they explore their views in more depth.

Evidence-informed decisions

In clinical practice, attention has focused on evidence-based medicine. Decisions about the management of a patient are influenced by evidence as to the most appropriate approach for the patient. Likewise, there has been a move to an evidence-based approach in medical education with a move away from a PHOG approach, where decisions about teaching are made based on:

Prejudices; **H**unches; **O**pinions; and **G**uesswork (Harden and Lilley, 2000).

The use of evidence-informed decisions in medical education has gained momentum. The BEME (Best Evidence in Medical Education) Collaboration (https://www.bemecollaboration.org/) was established in 1999 to promote a culture of evidence-informed teaching (Harden et al., 1999). By 2014, BEME was recognised not just as a minority pursuit but as a mainstream interest of many (Hammick, 2004). BEME systematic reviews have addressed a wide range of topics such as the use of high-fidelity simulations, the impact of early clinical experience, the features of effective faculty development programmes and the effectiveness of feedback in assessment.

Student scholars can review current education practices in the school in the light of available evidence as to what is effective. For example, are the ten evidence-based principles relating to the use of simulation (Motola et al., 2013) applied to how simulation is used in the school? Are the benefits that can be gained from the introduction of clinical experiences early in the curriculum (Dornan et al., 2006) realised in practice?

Evidence to support evidence-informed decisions can be found in:

- Published reports and recommendations for practice in the medical education literature in journals such as Medical Teacher, MedEdPublish, Medical Education, Academic Medicine, and Teaching and Learning in Medicine. In letters to the Editor of Medical Teacher, students have applied the principles described in published articles in the journal to situations in their own school
- Reviews of the available evidence as reported in the BEME and other systematic reviews
- Description by experts in the field of what they consider as a best practice as found in the AMEE Guides for the practising teacher and in Ottawa Consensus Statements with regard to best assessment practice

Students can be encouraged to engage with evidence from these sources by participating in, or by establishing their own, medical education journal clubs or seminar series to discuss research papers and their implications for practice within their school.

The student scholar as an innovator and agent for change

This is a time of change in medical education in response to alterations in public expectations, developments in medicine and the delivery of health care, and advances in educational approaches (Harden and Laidlaw, 2020). The student can play an important role in supporting and contributing to the implementation of new initiatives in the medical school. The student scholar should be a change mover and not just a recipient of change.

As Henry Miller (1966), Dean of Medicine at the University of Newcastle (UK), suggested all teachers, and we argue all students, have a responsibility for change:

> *It is useful occasionally to take a fresh look at a situation which we who are busily occupied in its day-to-day activities are often inclined to regard as immutable. In fact, of course, the present situation presents nothing more than a stage in an untidy historical process to which each generation must make its contribution, and effective change depends on continuing examination and criticism.*

Good ideas for change in medical education, it has been suggested (Harden and Lilley, 2018), may stagnate in a curriculum bureaucracy if this is committed to maintaining the status quo, either overtly or inadvertently. Fredrich Hess (2010) discussed

> *…repeated attempts to improve a fundamentally outdated, outmoded structure. Rather than explore and develop new structures, reformers pour their faith and resources into making the existing structure more effective. They tend to color safely within the lines – largely because those lines are so taken for granted that would-be reformers don't realize there is an alternative.*

Student scholars can help to ensure that an alternative approach to education, and what may be seen as a disruptive innovation, is given the attention it deserves and that new approaches to education are explored and developed. For example, the student-led Planetary Health Report Card audit of medical schools opens conversations about outcomes and skills for future doctors; medical schools' sustainability practices; and opportunities for community engagement to promote sustainability (Box 10.2). Students can also initiate change in the curriculum by reviewing and suggesting changes that lead towards a more diverse and inclusive curriculum. A group of 120 students at Queen's University in Canada reviewed 900 pieces of learning material related to dermatological conditions to identify the range of skin tones used. This highlighted a reliance on light skin tones and led to recommendations to revise the learning materials used (Rupnik, 2021).

Box 10.2 Student-led planetary health audit

https://phreportcard.org/

The Planetary Health Report Card is a student-driven, metric-based initiative to inspire planetary health and sustainable healthcare education engagement in medical schools. In addition to the inspiring expansion of medical school curricula, we hope to inspire medical schools to expand research efforts, engage with communities most affected by climate change and environmental injustice, support passionate medical students who are trying to organize around planetary health at the institutional level, and implement sustainable practices. A set of metrics in these five category areas allows students and faculty to conduct a needs assessment at their medical school.

The student as a researcher

Student engagement with research may be a formal part of the curriculum with the expectation that the student undertakes a research project, perhaps in collaboration with a member of staff, as an essential course requirement. Research is a prominent feature of intercalated degree programmes. There are often other opportunities for students to get involved as interns in ongoing research projects within medical schools or the broader university. For example, at the University of Edinburgh, students are invited as volunteers or interns to work with staff on rapid reviews of COVID-19 evidence to inform policymakers (UNCOVER: https://www.ed.ac.uk/usher/uncover). Students can approach staff to explore the potential opportunities for experience in research and such opportunities can be advertised online.

The student can play an important role in research in education. Such research is not simply about what works and what does not work; it is about understanding and illuminating why it works and the educational circumstances in which it works. As an actor in the process, students are well-placed to understand the problem being investigated and the solutions being proposed. In what ways, for example, may the flipped classroom be better than the traditional lecture, and how can it most effectively be included in the education programme? How can simulators and simulated patients be used to support rather than replace clinical teaching with patients? Students can help to extend an understanding of the education programme by engaging in research that contributes answers to such questions. Students can also join medical education research groups, for example, the MedEd Collaborative (Box 10.3).

Students may be involved in educational research in many ways, such as informing the questions to be asked, advising on the research design (for example, how students may respond to a survey request), and as peer researchers conducting surveys or interviews. The AMEE Guide 56 by Ringsted et al. (2011) provides a useful introduction to research in medical education and to the different approaches that may be adopted by students in this role.

Box 10.3   MedEd collaborative

https://www.mededcollaborative.org/about-us

Initiated in September 2020, the MedEd Collaborative is a national research group with the aim of promoting high-quality medical education research and audit amongst students and trainees.

In response to the disruption to medical education caused by COVID-19, there is a need for wide-scale robust medical education research and the generation of research capacity for the future. Trainee research collaboratives have demonstrated they can nurture the research skills of students and trainees while delivering high quality research outputs.

Our vision is to increase engagement of students and trainees in high-quality medical education research that informs practice. The MedEd Collaborative will engage students and trainees in medical education research by completing at least one national multicentre study per year.

Students can also engage in what is described as action research, studying their learning as a student. In action research, the student diagnoses a problem in practice, finds and implements solutions to the problem, and evaluates solutions in practice. Cohen and Manion (1980) have provided a useful description of action research:

Small scale intervention in the function of the real world and a close examination of the effects of such intervention. Action research is situational – it is concerned with diagnosing a problem in a specific context, it is usually (though not inevitably) collaborative – teams of researchers and practitioners work together on a project, it is participatory – team members themselves take part directly or indirectly by implementing the research and it is self-evaluative – modifications are continuously evaluated within the ongoing situation, the ultimate objective being to improve practice in some way or another (p. 186).

Box 10.4 gives an example of a student action research project.

The student scholar communicates about their experience

The student scholar shares their thoughts, experiences, and knowledge with other stakeholders. They can do this in a number of ways.

- Articles or letters published in the medical education literature
- Presentations (papers, posters, and workshops) at medical education conferences
- Presentations at curriculum or other education committee meetings locally or nationally
- Dissemination to other students within their school and in the wider medical student community
- Dissemination to other relevant stakeholders, for example, patient organisations

In Box 10.5, we present a student's reflections on their experience of communicating the findings from their research.

Box 10.4   Improving practice through action research

Von Pressentin et al. (2016) adopted an action research approach to improve work-based learning for Stellenbosch University's Longitudinal Integrated Clerkship (LIC). A participatory action research (PAR) approach was chosen because it allows researchers and participants to work together by reflecting on and changing their practice. A cooperative inquiry group (CIG) method (Mash and Meulenberg-Buskens, 2001), involving ten participants consisting of the students, clinician educators, and researchers, was used. Through a cyclical process of action and reflection, this group identified a teaching intervention. This cyclical process follows four steps repeated in an ongoing spiral of action (having an experience), observation (reviewing the experience), reflection (learning from the experience), and planning (based on new learning).

Box 10.5 Student case study: communicating research findings

10

A student reflects on making the connections needed to reach the right audiences, by Arthur Sebag, University of Glasgow

As a graduate entry student, I came into medicine with a pre-existing interest in drug harm reduction, through my involvement with the social enterprise Drugs and Me (https://drugsand.me). As I progressed through the course I was dismayed at its absence within the curriculum, compounded by negative attitudes towards people who use drugs, evidenced by the dehumanising language often used. Influencing the curriculum seemed like a great way to effect change, but it took me a long time to find purchase. After a lot of floundering, my fourth choice SSC provided the breakthrough. It was an opportunity to design a small pilot project and gather data. Rushing over winter break, I wrote up an application for ethical approval to run an online survey and a focus group to gauge student perception of recreational drug teaching.

I was able to generate interesting data, but that's when the real work starts – getting the right individuals to notice. I was lucky in that the lead for the block that contained the sole "alcohol and other drugs" week was my PBL facilitator. We struck up a discussion about helping her to review the content, but in between the pandemic and phase 3 "15 weeks of hell", this never moved forwards significantly.

I had a written-up article, so I submitted an abstract to a multi-disciplinary student journal. I didn't get the desired PubMed citation, but I found that networking with academics on the basis of getting advice for my paper was very effective. One of these connections got Drugs and Me in the Independent newspaper, and the other got me presenting to a working group of Scottish addiction specialists with the intent to expand the research nationally.

My top tip? Send a passionate email; people are very responsive to them.

Writing for publication

Students, as noted above, are making an increasing contribution to the published literature in medical education. A full description of the steps to producing a paper for publication and hints on getting it accepted is beyond the scope of this book; useful advice is given by Sharma and Ogle (2022) in their paper, *"Twelve Tips for students who wish to write and publish"*.

There are challenges for students in publishing their work, and staff can help by offering advice.

- Consider publication at an early stage: if there is an intention to publish the findings from a project, it is useful to ensure that the requirements to publish are considered in the planning of the project. For example, has ethical approval been sought and awarded?
- If publication is a strong motivator for students, staff can advise on the type of project that may be achievable given time and other resource constraints. For example, a scoping review may be more achievable for a short student project than a qualitative research study, given the requirement for ethical approval and the challenges associated with recruiting participants.
- Where there are open-access options, staff may be able to advise students on applying for any internal funds to support the costs incurred and schools may consider offering an annual award to support open-access publications.

- Students can also be reminded that academic publications are not always the best way to reach intended audiences. There are other forms of dissemination of research findings that engage with stakeholders outside of academia.

Contributing to an education conference

Scholarship can be demonstrated through a contribution to an education conference, such as the annual AMEE conference, which is attended by more than 300 students each year. Students can participate and make a short communication or poster presentation, contribute to the discussion in a plenary or symposium session from a student's perspective, and engage as a member of a student task force. In Box 10.6, we present an example of a student's experience of presenting at a virtual conference.

Some schools support a student's registration fees and travel costs incurred in participating in an education conference. We would encourage all schools to do this in order to create a more level playing field to ensure that there are no financial barriers to particular students having such opportunities.

Alternative methods of communication

Writing for publication and presenting at conferences may be appropriate modes of communicating research findings to academic and clinical audiences and can be interesting and beneficial experiences for student scholars. However, students may be engaged in research that is relevant to groups that may not usually attend such conferences, including other students, patients, those working in health-related voluntary sector organisations, and members of the public. It is useful, therefore, to consider the audience to whom you want to communicate your message and how best to reach that audience.

Box 10.6 Student case study: presenting at a conference

A student reflects on their experience of presenting at a virtual conference, by Siena I Hayes, Cardiff University Medical School

COVID-19 has had a profound impact on the opportunities available to medical students. I have attended virtual conferences but felt I didn't gain as much from them as I would at an in-person event due to communication and socialising being less fluid. Prior to the event, I was relieved I did not have to travel or spend extra on a hotel - however, the actual reality of a virtual conference was slightly disappointing. Whilst there were numerous opportunities to apply to conferences, I had little understanding of the difference between them, particularly regarding whether my research would be a good fit for their programme. I very much went with the approach of entering as many as I could, even if my paper was only tangentially related to the topic area of the conference. This meant I did receive numerous rejections, but as this is my first experience within the world of medical research, I saw it as a learning curve.

When the time came to present my accepted research, I presented my poster in my university bedroom to a blank screen, knowing numerous people were watching. It felt anti-climactic to not see the faces and human expressions we are normally greeted with at the end of a presentation. I think this has been a barrier for medical students, developing interests in research and opportunities in the future. Virtual conferences seem much less enticing with many choosing not to attend. Conferences and meetings are a chance to talk with like-minded people and spark interest in your work; much of this element is lost in virtual conferences.

Knowing who are the key stakeholders, or interested parties, in relation to research is important in shaping plans for dissemination. Identifying the relevant groups helps to be able to ensure that the messages reach the relevant people, are framed in a way that is meaningful for them and are communicated in a way that is accessible and engaging (Brownson et al., 2018). For example, if students conduct a research project that identifies problematic healthcare experiences among LGBTQIA+ students, they may want to communicate the findings to clinicians, but also to peers (medical students), to student well-being services, and to external organisations involved in LGBTQIA+ advocacy.

It is important to encourage students to engage with stakeholders when planning the dissemination of their research. There are also some tools available, for example, the Agency for Healthcare Research and Quality dissemination planning tool (https://www.ahrq.gov/sites/default/files/wysiwyg/professionals/quality-patient-safety/patient-safety-resources/resources/advances-in-patient-safety/vol4/planningtool.pdf).

Some suggestions for reaching a range of audiences include:

- *Event:* organising an event to share findings can be a useful way of engaging in a dialogue with relevant groups about the research findings (Hagan et al., 2017)
- *Social media:* can be very effective to share key messages and can be targeted to platforms used by particular groups, linking through existing networks
- *Blogs, videos, and podcasts:* can allow a slightly longer but still succinct summary of key messages and can be publicised via social media
- *Visual communication:* key messages can be effectively communicated visually, for example, by using infographics or cartoons

In Box 10.7, we present a student case study that reflects on the importance of involving patients in events for the British Undergraduate Society of Obstetrics and Gynaecology.

Box 10.7 Student case study: working with patients to develop extra-curricular activities

The experience of students organising events for the British Undergraduate Society of Obstetrics and Gynaecology, by Katrina Freimane, Queen's University Belfast and Molly Amira Kavanagh, Nottingham University (Events and Finance 2020-2022)

As we entered our roles as events officers for the British Undergraduate Society of Obstetrics and Gynaecology in Spring of 2021, we were aware that we were entering an already oversaturated virtual arena. We decided that a way to stand out and maximise our impact as a society would be to have patient representation in all our events. We wanted to create something that would be informative and engaging while helping to bridge the gap left by the cancelled placements due to Covid-19. We received excellent feedback about our patient speakers from the outset. The patient talks gave context and a sense of reality, alongside useful advice and information, which often helped bring the paired clinical speaker's talk to life.

It allowed us and our members to see the true impact of what we hope will be our future work, both positive and negative. It was heart-warming to hear about the significant effect a small act of kindness from a doctor can bring to a patient, and inspiring to see how respectful the dialogue was between the attendees and patients. We also did not shy

Continued

Box 10.7 Student case study: working with patients to develop extra-curricular activities—cont'd

away from patients who recounted times the profession had let them down; for example, in a webinar about pre-eclampsia where a patient recounted how many times she had been misdiagnosed. These were possibly the most useful stories of all, allowing us and the attendees to learn from the mistakes of others.

Whilst the positives will be taken forward and the negatives reflected on, as a committee we have felt empowered and more confident after hosting and attending these events. We hope that we have made some difference, even small, and will continue to prioritise patient voices in our activities. As hopeful future obstetricians and gynaecologists, we are aware of the speciality's marked history of patient neglect and abuse. This makes patient representation feel especially important to us, and we hope to continue to include patient representatives in our work going forward.

Conclusions

Recognising students as scholars has educational and personal benefits. Students can demonstrate scholarship in education by critically reflecting on their experiences in the education programme, applying an evidence-informed approach to examine practice in their school, contributing to innovating and introducing new approaches, engaging in research, and communicating their experiences to other stakeholders through suitable approaches including published papers, presentations at education conferences and other events, blogs, podcasts, and visual communication.

Students should be encouraged to use a scholarly approach when engaging with their different roles in the curriculum. The extent to which a scholar role is encouraged will vary from school to school and is likely to be related to how the school values teaching. As a scholar, students can be part of communities of staff and students (within their school and beyond) where scholarship is valued with new approaches to research and education adopted and facilitated by student engagement.

References

Boyer, E.L., 1990. Scholarship Reconsidered: Priorities of the Professoriate. Jossey-Bass, San Francisco, USA.

Brownson, R.C., Eyler, A.A., Harris, J.K., Moore, J.B., Tabak, R.G., 2018. Getting the word out: New approaches for disseminating publich health science. J. Public Health Manag. Pract. 24 (2), 102–111.

Cleland, J.A., Jamieson, S., Kusurkar, R.A., Ramani, S., Wilkinson, T.J., van Schalkwyk, S., 2021. Redefining scholarship for health professions education: AMEE Guide No. 142. Med. Teach. 43 (7), 824–838.

Cohen, L., Manion, L., 1980. Research Methods in Education. Croom Helm, London, UK.

Dornan, T., Littlewood, S.A., Margolis, A., Scherpbier, A., Spencer, J., Ypinazar, V., 2006. How can experience in clinical and community settings contribute to early medical education? A BEME systematic review. Med. Teach. 28 (1), 3–18.

Federal Way Public Schools, 2017. The Great Scholar vs. Student Debate | Q&A for Mr. FW. Federal Way Public Schools. https://www.federalwaymirror.com/opinion/the-great-scholar-vs-student-debate-qa-for-mr-fw/.

Hagan, T.L., Schmidt, K., Ackison, G.R., Murphy, M., Jones, J.R., 2017. Not the last word: Dissemination strategies for patient-centred research in nursing. J. Res. Nurs. 22 (5), 388–402.

Hammick, M., 2004. Take-home messages from AMEE 2004 in Edinburgh. Med. Teach. 26 (8), 739–742.

Harden, R.M., Crosby, J.R., Davis, M.H., Friedman, M., 1999. AMEE Guide No. 14: Outcome-based education: Part 5-From competency to meta-competency: A model for the specification of learning outcomes. Med. Teach. 21 (6), 546–552.

Harden, R.M., Laidlaw, J.M., 2012. Be FAIR to students: Four principles that lead to more effective learning. Med. Teach. 35 (1), 27–31.

Harden, R.M., Laidlaw, J.M., 2020. Essential Skills for a Medical Teacher (3rd ed). Elsevier, London, UK.

Harden, R.M., Lilley, P.M., 2000. Best evidence medical education: The simple truth. Med. Teach. 22 (2), 117–119.

Harden, R.M., Lilley, P., 2018. The Eight Roles of the Medical Teacher. Elsevier, London, UK.

Hess, F., 2010. The Same Thing Over and Over Again. Harvard University Press, Boston, Massachusetts, USA.

Jean, D., 2018. Dear Educators/Administrators: EVERY Student is a Scholar. Diverse Education. https://www.diverseeducation.com/students/article/15103485/dear-educators-administrators-every-student-is-a-scholar.

Mash, B., Meulenberg-Buskens, I., 2001. Holding it lightly': The co-operative inquiry group: A method for developing educational materials. Med. Educ. 35 (12), 1108–1114.

Motola, I., Devine, L.A., Chung, H.S., Sullivan, J.E., Issenberg, S.B., 2013. Simulation in healthcare education: A best evidence practical guide. AMEE Guide No. 82. Med. Teach. 35 (10), e1511–e1530.

Miller, H., 1966. Fifty years after Flexner. Lancet. 288 (7465), 647–654.

Palmer, Y.M., 2016. Student to scholar: learning experiences of international students. J. Int. Students. 6 (1), 216–240.

Ringsted, C., Hodges, B., Scherpbier, A., 2011. The research compass: An introduction to research in medical education: AMEE Guide no. 56. Med. Teach. 33 (9), 695–709.

Rupnik, C., 2021. Medical students review curriculum to improve racial representation in learning materials. The Queen's University Journal, Ontario, Canada. https://www.queensjournal.ca/story/2021-03-12/news/medical-students-review-curriculum-to-improve-racial-representation-in-learning-materials/.

Sharma, R.K., Ogle, H.L., 2022. Twelve tips for students who wish to write and publish. Med. Teach. 44 (4), 360–365.

von Pressentin, K.B., Waggie, F., Conradie, H., 2016. Towards tailored teaching: Using participatory action research to enhance the learning experience of Longitudinal Integrated Clerkship students in a South African rural district hospital. BMC Med. Educ. 16 (82).

11 Student participation in practice: some final thoughts

Student participation – an important development

Student participation and engagement in decisions relating to the education programme and in its delivery is an important item on today's agenda in medical education. As we discussed in Chapter 1, the concepts of student engagement, the student voice, and the student as a partner are important developments in medical education. The associated changing roles for the student are discussed in Chapter 2. In this final chapter we:

- Remind readers of the seven roles for the student, as discussed in Chapters 4–10, each with its own features and responsibilities.
- Review the benefits of student participation from the perspectives of the student, the teacher and the medical school.
- Explore the challenges for student participation from different perspectives.
- Describe the Student Participation Ladder, which represents the different levels and scope of student participation. Schools can determine their current position on the ladder and where they would like to be.
- Examine how student participation can be facilitated and the approaches that can be adopted to support this.
- Consider the future of student participation in the context of ongoing developments in medical education. We challenge the reader to imagine if what is thought to be impossible with regard to student participation is in fact possible.

The seven roles of the student

The roles of the student described in Figure 11.1 are:

- *The student as a professional:* demonstrating professionalism as a student doctor, as a learner, in relation to their health and well-being and with respect to civic responsibilities
- *The student as a facilitator of their learning:* a self-directed learner using tools such as a list of learning outcomes, a study guide, and a curriculum map to facilitate their own learning
- *The student as an information processor:* using a range of education strategies to make their processing of information effective and efficient

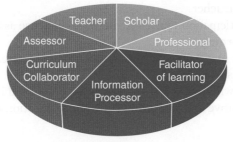

Figure 11.1 The seven roles of the student.

- *The student as curriculum collaborator:* evaluating the curriculum, impacting decisions through the curriculum committee and working with staff as a curriculum co-creator
- *The student as an assessor:* enhancing assessment decisions and with responsibility for self-assessment and peer assessment
- *The student as a teacher:* with responsibility for peer teaching, creating learning resources and peer mentorship
- *The student as a scholar:* reflecting on the education programme, applying an evidence-based approach, engaging in research and innovation and communicating their experience

The benefits of student participation

In Chapters 1 and 2, we introduce the benefits to be gained if there is greater involvement of the student in the design and implementation of the curriculum. In later chapters, the advantages gained from involving students in each role are explored further. The benefits include:

1. An improved learning experience for the student
   - A more authentic curriculum with improvements in the delivery of the education programme.
   - The curriculum becomes more student centred.
2. The personal development of the student
   - Students' engagement with the curriculum will contribute to the development of the student's professional identity and practice.
   - A wider range of learning outcomes is achieved including creativity, critical thinking, innovation, and negotiation skills.
3. Motivation of the student
   - The move towards the student as partner in the learning programme results in greater motivation for the student and more effective learning.
   - The student develops a stronger sense of belonging, mattering and ownership of the education programme.
   - A lasting relationship is developed between the student and the school with the student continuing to promote and support the school after graduation.

4. Benefits for the teacher
   - Student participation may constructively challenge assumptions about the teaching-learning process.
   - The teacher may gain a new excitement for and interest in teaching.
5. Benefits for the school
   - The school will benefit from all the above points and is encouraged to be more innovative and forward-looking in its education programme.

The challenges of student participation

Student participation may represent an important departure from established practice and is associated with challenges for the student, the teacher and the school. In previous chapters we discussed the challenges and barriers associated with student participation in each of the roles described and suggested ways to approach them. Later in this chapter, we discuss responding to the challenges in broader terms. Challenges to be considered include those related to:

1. *Students*
   - Students are transient and may be available to engage with the process only for a limited time.
   - Students may vary in their motivation or commitment, and this may change with the same student over time.
   - There may be conflicting priorities and tension arising from a student's personal study, other work/life commitments, and their available time to commit to the curriculum.
   - Students may experience an emotional burden as a result of engagement, particularly in relation to advocacy work.
   - Students may not believe that they have sufficient knowledge or skills to participate in decisions relating to the education programme.
2. *Teachers*
   - Teachers may feel threatened if the established hierarchy is challenged.
   - Teachers may not understand the different roles and how collaboration can work in practice with input from both student and teacher.
   - The collaboration with students may be time consuming and teachers may have other priorities that are more highly valued by the university.
3. *The process*
   - An investment of time is necessary, and it may be felt, by teachers or students, that this is not worth the effort.
   - The output of the process may be uncertain.
   - Existing power relations between the student and teacher can be difficult to realign.
   - There may not be funds to support initiatives, creating a barrier to some students' involvement, and so an inequity of opportunity among students.

4. *School governance*

- The procedures and governance arrangements within the school, including the hierarchal structure and the committee arrangements, may make the student's contribution difficult and tokenistic rather than meaningful.
- The culture and environment in the school may not be supportive of student participation, particularly if initiatives are seen as a fundamental departure from established approaches. Indeed, the term "student as partner" may seem too radical.

The student participation ladder

Views about student participation in the education programme are often polarised with some teachers believing that students should not have a role in managing and delivering the curriculum – "students are there to learn, teachers are there to teach" – while others embrace the involvement of students as partners in the education programme.

In the 1970s, '80s, and '90s, decisions about educational strategies were polarised with some for and others against strategies such as integration and problem-based learning. Rather than arguing for or against each strategy the SPICES model Harden et al. (1984) provided a tool to help the school constructively discuss where it should stand on each of the continua: student-/teacher-centred learning; problem-based/information-based; integrated/discipline-based; community-based/hospital-based; electives/uniform; systematic/opportunistic. In a similar way, in thinking about student participation, the question should not be whether a school should adopt student participation or not, but where should the school be on a continuum between no participation at one end and students in control of the programme at the other end. Both extremes are untenable.

Catherine Bovill (2020) in *Co-creating Learning and Teaching* described a ladder relating to students' role in curriculum design. There are many examples of ladder models to describe participation in other contexts (Arnstein, 1969). Such models are not intended to be prescriptive or to describe a linear sense of progression. Rather, the "ladder" is a simple metaphor to identify different positions along a continuum. We have adapted this model to apply to students' participation in the roles described in this book, as presented in Figure 11.2.

Steps in the ladder

The steps in the ladder are:

Step 0: No involvement of students. The school dictates the curriculum, and students' views are not sought on decisions about the curriculum or its implementation; students have no opportunities to evaluate their education programme. For example, students are not consulted concerning adopted educational methods such as the replacement of lectures with online learning resources.

Step 1: Review by students. Students are given the opportunity to review the education programme and identify its strengths and weaknesses. This is frequently done using evaluation questionnaires completed by students at the end of the course, as described in Chapter 7. The evaluation process, however, is frequently tokenistic, and the views expressed by students have limited impact on future curriculum planning. For example, questions related to educational methods and the use of new technologies are included in course evaluation questionnaires, but students' views are not acted upon in planning the programme for the following year.

Step 2: Consultation with students. The need to take students' views into account is recognised, and students are invited to contribute their perspectives at relevant meetings, for example at the curriculum committee. While their views are considered, students may not be involved in bringing about the necessary change or contributing to actions relating to the ongoing development of the

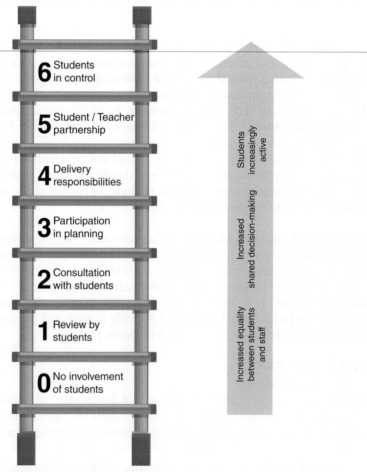

Figure 11.2 The student participation ladder. The six steps in the ladder are identified. A *side arrow* highlights the three trends as we move up the ladder.

education programme. For example, student representatives on the curriculum committee report the views of their peers that the number of lectures is excessive. There is agreement at the committee meeting that this should be addressed, but no agreement as to how it should be and how students can contribute to the resolution of the problem.

Step 3: Participation in planning. Planning for the implementation of changes agreed upon with regard to the education programme is carried out in collaboration with students. For example, following the discussion of the student concern relating to the number of lectures, the decision is taken jointly by staff and students on the curriculum committee to introduce a revised lecture schedule for Years 1 and 2, following a content review by module leads.

Step 4: Responsibilities for delivery. Students are given specific responsibilities in relation to the education programme. For example, the student anatomy society is encouraged to offer peer tutorials, as described in Chapter 9, for content no longer considered core following the revision of the lecture schedule.

Step 5: A partnership. This step represents a negotiated education programme with collaboration and joint decisions by staff and students. As described in Chapter 7 in relation to curriculum co-creation, there is a sense of connectedness which allows staff and students to collectively shoulder the responsibility for the development and implementation of the education programme. For example, following the discussion of the students' concerns related to the number of lectures, a group of students work collaboratively with module leads to review and suggest changes to content and modes of delivery.

Step 6: Students in control. As described in Chapter 5 in the example of *The Independent Project* (Wehmeyer and Zhao, 2020), the students are in control of the education programme. While staff may be involved in an advisory role, the responsibility and final decisions for the content, expected learning outcomes, education strategies, and teaching and learning methods rest with the students.

How the seven roles are reflected in the steps of the Student Participation Ladder is illustrated with the examples in Table 11.1. The student roles as we describe in the earlier chapters are wide-ranging, and we have chosen only examples for illustrative purposes.

As we move up the ladder, students are increasingly actively involved and there is a greater extent of shared decision-making, moving towards a partnership between staff and students. The nature of the students' participation and the extent and impact of this across the curriculum increases. We consider the bottom of the ladder, where there is no student involvement, as untenable in the delivery of a quality medical education programme. The intention of the model is not to propose that all schools should or could be at the top of the ladder in all aspects of their work.

Table 11.1 Examples of the seven student roles as they relate to each of the steps in the student participation ladder

Step	Professional	Facilitator of Learning
6 Students in control	Students are given control over aspects of the curriculum relating to their civic professionalism	Students have responsibility for facilitating their own learning and choosing education strategies and learning opportunities best suited to their needs
5 Student/ Teacher partnership	A working group with a student and a teacher as co-chairs is established with the remit of exploring students' civic professionalism	A group of students and staff work together to produce a joint report with guidance for staff on writing learning outcomes and advice for students on how to use learning outcomes to facilitate their learning
4 Delivery responsibilities	Students are asked to prepare a briefing paper on community activities in other medical schools for consideration at a future meeting	Students are given the task of producing a curriculum map for the module with the learning outcomes embedded and related to available learning opportunities
3 Participation in planning	At a curriculum committee meeting staff and students agree to invite the university community engagement team to the next meeting to explore students' possible involvement in community initiatives	It is agreed that there is a problem with how the learning outcomes are specified and that the way in which the learning outcomes are stated and represented in a curriculum map should be reviewed
2 Consultation with students	Student representatives are given the opportunity to raise their concerns at a meeting of the curriculum committee which they are invited to attend, but no action is taken	In a yearly committee meeting, student representatives elaborate on the need for further information on what they should be learning
1 Review by students	In a programme evaluation questionnaire, students express concerns about the limited opportunities to develop civic professionalism	At an end of course evaluation, students complain that managing their own learning is difficult as the expected learning outcomes as stated are not clear
0 No involvement of students	Students' views on professionalism are not sought	Students have no opportunities to discuss their role as facilitators of their own learning

Table 11.1 Examples of the seven student roles as they relate to each of the steps in the student participation ladder—cont'd

Step	Information processor	Curriculum collaborator
6 Students in control	Students collectively determine the policies and practices that will make information processing effective and efficient	Students independently prepare a revised curriculum
5 Student/ Teacher partnership	A paper is produced jointly by staff and students which sets out the school's policy and practices with regard to supporting students' information processing	A working group co-chaired by staff and students is set up to create learning opportunities which address the gaps identified relating to LGBTQIA+ health
4 Delivery responsibilities	Students are asked to prepare a set of guidelines for students and teachers on an agreed information processing strategy - the use of question banks	Based on the findings of an audit, students are asked to develop proposals for a curriculum revision relating to LGBTQIA+ health
3 Participation in planning	As a result of student consultation, staff and students agree to a list of recommended strategies	It is agreed that an audit of the curriculum should be undertaken to identify where LGBTQIA+ issues are discussed and where there are opportunities for further inclusion
2 Consultation with student	A survey is sent to students to identify the range of information-processing strategies that students use	The issue is discussed by staff and students at the Equality, Diversity, and Inclusion committee and the need to review the LGBTQIA+ content of the curriculum is agreed
1 Review by students	Students report that additional guidance is needed on how they can best manage the increasing amount of information provided to them	A group of students send an email to the Programme Director noting the lack of attention given in the curriculum to LGBTQIA+ health
0 No involvement of students	Students are not involved in discussions as to how they can best process information	Students are not involved in curriculum development

Continued

Table 11.1 Examples of the seven student roles as they relate to each of the steps in the student participation ladder—cont'd

Step	Assessor	Teacher	Scholar
6 Students in control	Students have control over elements of the assessment process with greater importance attached to peer- and self-assessment	Students independently instigate a peer-teaching programme	Students take responsibility for creating research opportunities and for disseminating their research projects
5 Student/ Teacher partnership	The overall assessment policy described in the school's assessment PROFILE (Chapter 8) is agreed upon jointly by staff and students	Staff and students work jointly to agree to the principles for planning and delivery of a peer-teaching programme	Students and staff work together to develop an annual student research conference
4 Delivery responsibilities	Students are asked to review the rubric that has been developed by the assessment committee and to suggest revisions	A programme of peer teaching is introduced, and students are invited to serve as peer tutors	Students involved in research identify the available opportunities and the support required for the dissemination of their research findings
3 Participation in planning	It is agreed that there should be further discussion and a process prepared for students to work with staff in addressing the problem	It is agreed that a teaching skills curriculum should be developed and opportunities for peer teaching within a module and clinical settings identified	To support the students' role in research, a paid internship programme is proposed where students can work alongside research teams
2 Consultation with student	The assessment committee invites students to attend a meeting to discuss a possible mismatch between curriculum learning outcomes and the assessment programme	There is a discussion between staff and students at the curriculum committee that teaching and learning skills should be included in the curriculum and opportunities for students to serve as teachers offered	At the school research committee, student representatives are invited to join a discussion about the students' role in research
1 Review by students	In a programme evaluation students complain that there is a mismatch between the assessment methods and the expected learning outcomes	In a programme evaluation, students report that there is no training or opportunities for gaining experience as teachers within the curriculum	At a meeting of the Medical Students' Council, students raised a concern that there are few opportunities for them to engage in research
0 No involvement of students	Students are not involved in issues related to the planning and implementation of assessment	Students are not involved as teachers	Students have no opportunities to discuss their role as scholars

We hope, however, that the model will encourage students and staff to reflect on their school's position on the ladder. It is likely that each school will be positioned at different points in relation to the different student roles we have discussed in this book. For example, a school may already actively engage students as teachers through a well-established peer teaching programme, organised by students, with support from staff where appropriate. In this respect, the school may be at level 4 or 5 on the ladder. However, the same school may be at level 2 or 3 in relation to other student roles.

The ladder model can be used to facilitate discussion between students and staff with regard to the nature and extent of student participation in planning and implementing the education programme. It can help to clarify in the context of a medical school, the implications for the seven student roles described in this book. This may not always be an easy process: with some of the roles, there may be clear agreement as to where the school lies on the model, what further student participation would mean, and how this can be achieved. However, in other areas, tensions may exist, and there is a risk that existing hierarchies may implicitly or explicitly limit the nature or extent of change (as discussed later in the chapter). It is likely that as schools seek to move to the higher levels on the ladder such tensions may be more apparent. Moving towards meaningful partnerships (5) or student control (6) may be disruptive and may indeed require some fundamental rethinking of core aspects of the education programme. Below we offer some suggestions to help facilitate the discussions.

Facilitation of student participation

The development of student participation can be facilitated by:

- Adoption of a collaborative approach
- Initial appraisal of existing student participation in the school
- Familiarisation of staff and students with the concept of student participation
- Selection of an initial area for development
- Extending student participation and moving up the ladder
- Responding to the challenges of student participation

Adoption of a collaborative approach

Key to student participation in the education programme is a meaningful collaboration of the stakeholders, including, but not limited to, teaching staff, administration, deans, associate deans and curriculum leaders, and importantly the students. Collaboration is essential given that there may be divergent views as to the value of student involvement in the programme. It may help to set up a working group with staff and students as members and with a student engagement champion and a student as co-chairs. Such a group would have the potential to act as an exemplar of effective partnership working. Spending the time to make sure the group works well and represents the school's vision for enhancing student participation is important. This may involve:

- Discussion of expectations and ways of working
- Clarity on the roles within the group to avoid the students' roles being tokenistic
- Creation of appropriate options for group members to anonymously communicate concerns or suggestions about the working of the group
- Establishment of a process for remediation of disparate views that the group cannot resolve
- Payment to student members to compensate for their time and acknowledgement of staff contribution within workload models (or other methods of acknowledging such work)

The remit of the working group can be to determine the school's student participation strategy and:

- Establish a process of consultation with students and staff on student participative roles in the education programme
- Recommend where the school should aspire to be on the Student Participation Ladder and identify the necessary action to make this possible
- Identify ways to communicate the benefits of student participation and why the school should move in this direction
- Address questions about student participation in medical school such as:
  - Where should student participation be prioritised?
  - How can students be recognised and rewarded?
  - What staff training programme is required?
  - How will developments in the field be supported?
  - What changes, if any, are required in the school's governance and committee structure?
  - With whom should the responsibility lie for the necessary further action?

Initial appraisal of existing student participation

A useful initial step in developing student participation is an audit of, and consultation on, the current forms of student involvement in the school, reflecting on any successes, identifying where there is room for improvement and suggestions for further actions.

The provision of opportunities for both staff and students to contribute their views at this initial stage is essential. It is likely that a range of consultation approaches, including surveys, open meetings, and voting tools, may be necessary to be inclusive and reach as many people as possible. Brooman et al. (2015) described the value of focus groups in gaining a different perspective

> Using focus groups, we gained critical insight into how students received
> the first redesign in which we made mistakes. The student voice clarified,
> challenged and re-defined our approach to curriculum development. We found
> a better way to listen, and a value in doing so.

The information gathered can be used to gauge, from the different perspectives of students and staff, where the school lies on the Student Participation Ladder and where there are strengths and weaknesses relating to the seven roles described in this book. This consultation process may highlight shared views as well as points of difference and potential tensions.

Familiarisation of staff and students with the concept of student participation

In the exploration of student participation and the school's position on the participation ladder, it is helpful to ensure that teachers and students understand the rationale for student participation in the education programme, including the different approaches to the student's involvement as described in Chapters 4–10 and the benefits that can result as highlighted above.

Approaches to raising awareness about the changing roles of students and the benefits of student involvement should be discussed (with staff and students) and may include:

- The provision of case studies and examples of student participation in practice. The student reflections in this book can be used as illustrative examples to help students propose their own experiences or to encourage staff to gather experiences from their students.
- A range of communication tools such as infographics, posters, and video clips
- School-based workshops or webinars
- Suggested readings from educational journals
- Supporting staff and students' participation at medical education conferences where student participation is being discussed

Selection of an initial area for development

Assuming that a decision is taken to develop the level of student participation within the education programme, the question to be asked is how to proceed. Rather than an overambitious programme involving all areas of the curriculum, it may be more constructive to select one or more areas for particular attention. This may show how students can have an immediate impact and demonstrate the value and feasibility of the approach in the local context.

The initial consultation is likely to have identified priority areas that can then be discussed within the group. The seven roles of the student discussed in this book can be used to identify foci for activities. Examples include:

- Curriculum review of service learning opportunities (the student as a professional)
- Audit of student workload (the student as a facilitator of their own learning)

- Review of the use of lectures for student learning (the student as an information processor)
- Instigation of a student curriculum board (the student as a curriculum collaborator)
- Review of feedback processes (the student as an assessor)
- Development of peer observation of teaching (the student as a teacher)
- Support for a student conference (the student as a scholar)

Extending student participation and moving up the ladder

Following successful student participation in one area of the curriculum, maintaining the change and extending student involvement to other areas may run into difficulties with the initial change remaining isolated. As noted by Brasof (2018) (Box 11.1), an *organisational improvement paradox* tends to emerge when the student and the educator's sphere of influence is limited to the creators of the initiative. For the innovation to be successful, collaboration and unified action by all the stakeholders is necessary, and the school's culture and governance must be prepared to accept the change.

It is important to track changes across the programme to ensure a holistic awareness of student participation initiatives. Initiatives focused on specific curricular areas may be conducted by discrete groups, and there may be a benefit in establishing a form of reporting of activities or conducting an annual audit to maintain momentum in the enhancement work as a whole.

Consideration needs to be given to the impact of the increased student participation in the education programme, the benefits that derive from this in relation to improving the overall curriculum, the impact on a student's experience as a learner, and the additional benefits to staff and students of partnership work. Keeping students and staff informed of developments is also an important part of the wider student engagement strategy and will help to create a sense of connection with the work being undertaken.

Box 11.1 The organisational improvement paradox

An 'organisational improvement paradox' occurs when positive outcomes in one part of the organisation do happen but they fail to translate into gains elsewhere, which is frequently the case for student voice work (Brasof, 2018).

The organisational improvement paradox posits change is limited in terms of both impact and sustainment because implementers believe the efficacy of their work will spontaneously result in a spread. But without considering established organizational behaviours, structures, and processes, several hurdles for widening impacts can isolate change work.

The solution to this paradox resides in linkage theory (Goodman, 2000), the pathways that help connect activity, events and outcomes between change work to multiple levels of an organisation.

The involvement of students in many of the roles we have discussed in the book has the potential to disrupt traditional hierarchies in education, and as such may meet explicit or implicit resistance. In schools where the leadership team supports such an approach, it is likely that the path to change will be smoother, and any issues more easily raised and addressed. However, where that support is absent, students can still be agents of change and staff can support this, as champions of student participation in the programme.

Responding to the challenges

The challenges associated with student participation are described earlier in this chapter. These should be discussed when developing the core principles of student participation initiatives and partnership working and issues are likely to arise during the process. This reinforces the need to have an open and honest approach to working with students, to allow discussion and resolution of any problems as they arise. It may be useful to develop a student participation policy to establish expectations on ways of working collaboratively. While each initiative may have different requirements, it is important to establish agreement on the core principles. This could form part of the remit of the working group, if established, or be agreed upon following a consultation with staff and students.

In Chapter 1, we discussed the meaning of "partnership" in the context of student engagement. In some instances, responsibility for the initiative may be handed over to the students, for example, in the development of peer observation of a teaching scheme. At other times, it may be more appropriate for staff to take a lead or to distribute responsibility evenly between staff and students.

It is important to address explicitly the distribution of responsibility and power and the potential challenges this may present, and this can also be a constructive part of the process.

> I believe we should start by seeking the best out of both parties for the task at hand. Either way, viewing barriers such as power dynamics as opportunities to improve partnerships, rather than as roadblocks, is the first step (Kapadia, 2020).

It may also be useful to consider the values of partnership working, as a way to frame student participation initiatives

> Openness; trust and honesty; agreed shared goals and values; and regular communication between the partners" (QAA 2013, p. 3).

As suggested above in relation to the working group, it may be useful to have anonymous feedback opportunities and a process for remediating any disputes within the collaborative partnerships. This may help mitigate the risk of slipping back into pre-existing hierarchies where students' views are given less weight.

The future of student participation

There have been exciting developments in medical education with more authentic curricula, greater collaboration locally and internationally, fundamental changes in assessment and greater use of technology including virtual and augmented reality, online learning, and simulation. Technical developments have been associated with a better understanding of the psychology of learning and how students can be helped to achieve clearly articulated learning outcomes.

Wider social changes also demand ongoing changes in how medical students are educated. The Lancet report, *Health Professionals for a New Century: Transforming Education to Strengthen Health Systems in an Interdependent World* (Frenk et al., 2010), identified the most pressing global health challenges and noted that

> *Professional education has not kept pace with these challenges, largely because of fragmented, outdated, and static curricula that produce ill-equipped graduates.*

In looking to the future of medical education, student participation will be an important contributor to bringing about the changes in medical education required to ensure our graduates meet the needs of the communities they serve. In the 40th anniversary issue of Medical Teacher (October 2018), six leaders in medical education described their visions for the future of the medical school. They highlight the importance of student participation.

Hays (2018) argued that in the school of the future, governance and administration will require student participation in programme design and evaluation and student participation in programme management. Students will participate in decision-making about most aspects of the programme. A move from the student as a client to the student as a partner was described by Harden (2018) as one of the ten key features of the future medical school. The student will have a big impact on the education programme including curriculum planning, the creation of learning resources to support adaptive learning, the appointment of staff and the selection of students.

Rath et al. (2018) argued

> *There is a valuable partnership to be forged with students as we reimagine the future of medical training. The students are, in many ways, ahead of their institutions in sensing the future…Simply put, they want to direct their own educational content and experience.*

Hamdy (2018) pointed out that change in how we educate our students is a "wicked problem". Some aspects of the changes to student roles that we have described in this book may be relatively straightforward, and others, that are more disruptive and require deeper change, may indeed be wicked problems that will be difficult, but necessary to resolve. The difference between a simple change and a more challenging one will depend on the local context and where along the continuum a school or wider community of medical educators is currently placed.

Imagine if the impossible isn't

In *"Open to Think"*, Dan Pontefract (2018) argued that we need to slow down, think creatively, and make better decisions. We need to "Dream, decide, and do." Our hope is that *The Changing Role of Medical Students* will stimulate you to dream about how staff and students can work together in your school, to decide what you will do, and to do it.

We need to be innovative and think creatively, as noted by Hays (2018).

> *Most new medical schools tend to follow convention pathways, developing similar programs that provide similar student experiences, often as the 'safe' pathway to being accepted by potential applicants, the profession and accreditation bodies.*

We need, as proposed by Frederic Hess (2010), to colour outside of the lines.

> *Repeated attempts to improve a fundamentally outdated outmoded structure. Rather than explore and develop new structures, reformers pour their faith and resources into making the existing structure more effective. They tend to colour safely within the lines – largely because those lines are so taken for granted that would-be reformers don't realize there is an alternative.*

While we cannot be certain about the future of medical education, student participation in planning and implementing the education programme should be part of our plan.

> *While we can't know for sure what the future will be, we need to envision and plan medical education in order to help it evolve to meet future needs. A wider range of possibilities need to be considered for the unknowables of the future so we can 'Boldly go where no one has gone before' (Rourke, 2018).*

Developing student participation will not be easy. In *Future Driven*, David Guerin (2017) suggested

> *The best solutions aren't microwave friendly. They come through deeper thinking. They come by shifting perspective. Do the hard work of challenging the status quo. Ponder the deeper questions and look at the world in new and interesting ways.*

A final thought on the implementation of student participation approaches. Wayne Hodgins (2005), a future strategist, challenges readers to engage with an idea when it appears difficult or even impossible.

> *This future is ours for the choosing if we can muster the courage to ignite the transformation from vision to reality by simply imagining that this bright future is now possible and begin shaping its design and implementation. The trick is that it will take all of us to imagine, design, and build. If you can imagine this previously impossible dream now, you are already part of the solution.*

The challenge for all of our readers is for you to imagine the future with greater student participation and to play a part in making this happen.

References

Arnstein, S.A., 1969. A ladder of citizen participation. J. Am. Plann. Assoc. 35 (4), 216–224.

Bovill, C., 2020. Co-creating Learning and Teaching: Towards Relational Pedagogy in Higher Education. Critical Publishing, Essex, UK.

Brasof, M., 2018. Using linkage theory to address the student voice organizational improvement paradox. J. Ethical Educ. Leadersh. (S1), 44–65.

Brooman, S., Darwent, S., Pimor, A., 2015. The student voice in higher education curriculum design: Is there value in listening? Innov, Educ. Teach. Int. 52 (6), 663–674.

Frenk, J., Chen, L., Bhutta, Z.A., Cohen, J., Crisp, N., Evans, T., Fineberg, H., Garcia, P., Ke, Y., Kelley, P., 2010. Health professionals for a new century: Transforming education to strengthen health systems in an interdependent world. Lancet. 376, 1923–1958.

Goodman, P.S., 2000. Missing organizational linages: Tools for cross-level research. Sage, Thousand Oaks, Canada, USA.

Guerin, D., 2017. Future Driven: Will Your Students Thrive in an Unpredictable World? Self-Published.

Hamdy, H., 2018. Medical College of the future: from informative to transformative. Med. Teach. 40 (10), 986–989.

Harden, R.M., 2018. Ten key features of the future medical school – not an impossible dream. Med. Teach. 40(10), 1010–1015.

Harden, R.M., Sowden, S., Dunn, W.R., 1984. Educational strategies in curriculum development: The SPICES model. Med. Educ. 18 (4), 284–297.

Hays, R., 2018. Establishing a new medical school: A contemporary approach to personalizing medical education. Med. Teach. 40 (10), 990–995.

Hess, F.M., 2010. The Same Thing Over and Over: How School Reformers Get Stuck in Yesterday's Ideas. Harvard University Press, Boston, USA.

Hodgins, W., 2005. Into the future of me-learning: Everyone learning … imagine if the impossible isn't!. In: Masie, E. (Ed.), Learning Rants, Raves, and Reflections: A Collection of Passionate and Professional Perspectives. Wiley, New Jersey, USA. pp. 243–290.

Kapadia, S.J., 2020. Perspectives of a 2nd-year medical student on 'Students as Partners' in higher education – What are the benefits, and how can we manage the power dynamics? Med. Teach. 43 (4), 478–479.

Pontefract, D., 2018. Open to Think: Slow Down, Think Creatively and Make better Decisions Figure 1 Publishing, Vancouver, Canada.

Rath, V.L., Mazotti, L., Wilkes, M.S., 2018. A framework to understand the needs of the medical students of the future. Med. Teach. 42 (8), 922–928.

Rourke, J., 2018. What does the future hold? No one knows for sure... Med. Teach. 40 (10), 980–981.

The Quality Assurance Agency for Higher Education. UK Quality Code for Higher Education. QAA, Gloucester, UK.

Wehmeyer, M., Zhao, Y., 2020. Teaching Students to Become Self-Directed Learners. ASCD, Alexandria, Virginia, USA.

INDEX

Note: Page numbers followed by "*f*" indicate figures, "*t*" indicate tables, and "*b*" indicate boxes.